Pterygium Surgery

Congxiang Wang • Shaowei Li
Editors

Pterygium Surgery

Springer

PMPH
PEOPLE'S MEDICAL PUBLISHING HOUSE

Editors
Congxiang Wang
Changsha Aier Eye Hospital
Changsha, China

Shaowei Li
Beijing Aier Intech Eye Hospital
Beijing, China

ISBN 978-981-99-6845-9 ISBN 978-981-99-6843-5 (eBook)
https://doi.org/10.1007/978-981-99-6843-5

Jointly published with People's Medical Publishing House, PR of China

This Springer imprint is published by the registered company Springer Nature Singapore Pte Ltd.
The registered company address is: 152 Beach Road, #21-01/04 Gateway East, Singapore 189721, Singapore

Paper in this product is recyclable.

Preface

Pterygium is a degenerative conjunctival disease with an unknown aetiology and may be related to ultraviolet (UV) exposure, genetic factors, and dry and dusty environments. Clinically, pterygium is divided into three types: primary pterygium, recurrent pterygium, and pseudopterygium. The main clinical symptoms of pterygium include dry eye, eye itchiness, eye redness, foreign body sensation, photophobia, and blurred vision, although the symptoms are not specific. In severe cases, pterygium may involve the central part of the cornea, with a decline in or complete loss of vision. Recently, the number of pterygium patients with cosmetic concerns has gradually increased in China. Up till now, no medication is available for pterygium, and surgery is the only effective treatment.

Improving pterygium surgery has been a long and arduous process. Postoperative pterygium recurrence remains a clinical hurdle. To prevent pterygium recurrence, researchers have applied many therapeutic methods, such as antimetabolites, β radiation, and YAG laser resection, which can reduce but not completely eliminate the recurrence risk. Furthermore, surgeons are facing higher demands from patients to improve postoperative cosmetic outcomes.

In the past 10 years, we have been using the modified PERFECT surgical procedure to treat more than 15,000 cases of primary pterygium and different degrees of recurrent pterygium. No serious complications have been noted post-surgery, with a low recurrence rate, and the cosmetic outcomes have been satisfactory. In this book, we systematically summarize our clinical experience and cite many studies in the literature with the hope of providing our clinical peers with a reference guide.

My sincere thanks go to Mr. Yao Zhao from International Communication and Cooperation Department, Aier Eye Hospital Group who spare no efforts to organize and move forward the whole publication project of this English edition.

We sincerely thank Professor Xuguang Sun from the Aier Keratoconus Institute for his gracious encouragement and help with editing this book. When Professor Sun learned about our unique pterygium surgical approach in our hospital, he immediately suggested that we should write a book to systematically convey our surgical and clinical experiences to our peers. He also vigorously supported us in conducting retrospective research and prospective multicentre studies as our modified surgical method can be verified by evidence-based research.

We sincerely thank Professor Hansheng Liu, Deputy Director of the Medical Management Center of the Aier Eye Hospital Group, and Mr. Ziwen Huang of the Human Resources Center of the Aier Eye Hospital Group and the Aier School of Management for editing the surgical videos in this book. We express our gratitude to Dr. Ding Lin, President of Changsha Aier Eye Hospital, and all the operating room staff at Changsha Aier Eye Hospital and the Department of Special Examination for their generous help.

We thank Dr. Jun Chen, Dr. Qiao Yu, and Dr. Guihua Zou from the Department of Cornea and Ophthalmology of Changsha Aier Eye Hospital for their help with collecting information and for providing postoperative patient photos. Finally, we are especially grateful to all the patients who cooperated with us during treatment.

Changsha Aier Eye Hospital, Changsha, China Congxiang Wang
September 6, 2022
Beijing Aier Intech Eye Hospital, Beijing, China Shaowei Li

Contents

Part I
Basic Knowledge

Chapter 1
Epidemiology

Shaowei Li and Kuanshu Li

Pterygium is a common disease of the ocular surface with a long history. An Indian scholar, Susruta, first described pterygium and its surgical treatment in approximately 1000 BC. Through research by dozens of generations of ophthalmologists, Chakradatta et al. again described pterygium in detail and proposed treatment methods in 1060 AD.

Pterygium is **defined** by **a** triangular, wing-shaped, degenerative, fibrovascular, hyperplastic tissue growing from the bublo conjunctival through the corneal limbus into the cornea [1]. The term "pterygium" was given because of its "insect wing-like" appearance. Pterygium is the most common disease of the ocular surface. In addition to eye discomfort symptoms such as foreign body sensation, dryness, and redness of the eye, pterygium significantly affects the aesthetic appearance of the eye, and severe pterygium can lead to blindness and eyeball movement restriction.

1.1 Section 1: Prevalence and Incidence

1.1.1 Prevalence

Prevalence is the proportion of a population newly or previously diagnosed with a disease in a particular period. The reported prevalence of pterygium varies markedly among a number of recent studies, which might be attributable to three main reasons. First, the aetiology and pathogenesis of pterygium have not been fully

S. Li (✉)
Beijing Aier Intech Eye Hospital, Beijing, China
e-mail: lishaowei@aierchina.com

K. Li
Changsha Aier Eye Hospital, Changsha, China

C. Wang, S. Li (eds.), *Pterygium Surgery*,
https://doi.org/10.1007/978-981-99-6843-5_1

revealed. Second, many factors may influence the prevalence. Third, due to these studies had different designs, subjects, and sample sizes between the studies.

In 2018, Rezvan et al. [2] conducted a meta-analysis of the prevalence of pterygium that included 68 studies. They concluded that the global average prevalence was 12%, with the lowest regional prevalence was 0.07% and the highest regional was 53%. In a meta-analysis conducted by Yang et al. [3] in 2019 that included 36 studies, According to the prevalence of pterygium among people aged 40 and older in China was 13.4% between 1990 and 2016. Song et al. [4] reported that the prevalence of pterygium was 9.84% that should approximately 109 million pterygium patients were between 15 and 84 years of age in China in 2010.

The factors influencing the pterygium prevalence include the following:

1. **Geographic location**: Because the occurrence of pterygium is closely related to ultraviolet (UV) radiation, the prevalence of pterygium varies with latitude and altitude. Particularly, the prevalence of pterygium is relatively higher in areas between 40°N and 40°S, which are collectively referred to as the "pterygium belt" [5].

   The reported prevalence of pterygium in China varies markedly due to China's vast geographical span, ranging from 2.9% among people over 40 years of age in rural Beijing [6] to 33.0% among people over 50 years of age in rural Guangdong [7].

   Song et al. [4] conducted a study on the prevalence of pterygium in China and found that the number of patients with pterygium was lowest in the Tibet Autonomous Region (population approximately 210,000) and largest in Guangdong Province (population approximately 12.29 million). The prevalence of pterygium was lowest in Heilongjiang Province (4.16%) and highest in Hainan Province (18.02%). The study concluded that the prevalence of pterygium was higher in low-latitude areas than in high-latitude areas and was not correlated with longitude.

   Liu et al. [8] analysed the geographical distribution of pterygium and revealed that except for the area between 20° and 30° latitude, the prevalence of pterygium increased with decreasing latitude, a finding that may be related to strong solar radiation at low latitudes. However, the cause of the high prevalence of pterygium in the area between 20° and 30° latitude remains unclear (Table 1.1).

   In addition, the prevalence of pterygium is related to altitude. Lu et al. [9] investigated the area above 3000 m in Zeku County (also known as Zêkog County) in Qinghai Province and found that 323 of 2229 Tibetans had pterygium; the prevalence rate was 14.49%. In comparison, the prevalence was 10.53% in

Table 1.1 The prevalence of pterygium at different latitudes

Latitude	Prevalence of pterygium (%)
0–10°	14.80
10–20°	13.40
20–30°	19.30
30–40°	5.90
40–50°	4.10

Shandong Province at similar latitudes [10], indicating that the prevalence of pterygium is higher in high-altitude areas than in low-altitude areas.

2. **Age**: Pterygium is more common in elderly populations; however, it can also occur in younger people (10–30 years of age). Most patients with primary pterygium at young age have family history. The prevalence of pterygium increases with age. In a meta-analysis of the prevalence of pterygium among people aged 40 and older in China, Yang et al. reported that the prevalence increased significantly with age, except for the population aged 80 years and older [3] (Table 1.2). A global meta-analysis similarly showed that the prevalence of pterygium increased significantly with age: 0.3% in the 10- to 20-year-old age group and 19.5% in the ≥80-year-old age group [2] (Table 1.3).
3. **Sex:** Whether the occurrence of pterygium is related to sex is still controversial. In Hebei Province in China, the prevalence rates of pterygium are 7.8% among men and 5.7% among women [11]. A study in Iran showed that the prevalence rates of pterygium were 13% among women and 18% among men [12].
4. **Race**: Whether the occurrence of pterygium is related to race remains controversial. Nemesure et al. [13] found that the prevalence of pterygium was lower among white people than among ethnic groups with darker skin colours. In an epidemiological study conducted by Ang et al. [14] with Malaysian, Indian, and Chinese individuals living in Singapore, the prevalence of pterygium was 10.1% overall in the region and was significantly higher among Malaysian individuals (15.5%) than among Indian (7.0%) and Chinese (7.0%) individuals. Despite their darker skin colour, the prevalence of pterygium was not higher among Indian individuals than among Malaysian and Chinese individuals, indicating that in addition to race, other factors (e.g., genetic factors, age, sex, outdoor

Table 1.2 Meta-analysis of the prevalence of pterygium among different age groups in China

Age (years)	Number of studies included	Prevalence of pterygium	I^2 value (%)
≥40	15	8.8%	99.24
≥50	27	13.2%	99.23
≥60	26	16.7%	99.33
≥70	25	19.2%	95.93
≥80	19	15.4	99.74

Table 1.3 Global meta-analysis of the prevalence of pterygium among different age groups

Age (years)	Number of patients included	Prevalence of pterygium (%)	I^2 value (%)
10–20	2922	0.3	80.9
20–29	1829	1.6	87.6
30–39	4660	5.6	98.1
40–49	20,575	7.8	97.1
50–59	40,918	11.2	98.2
60–69	41,783	16.7	98.8
70–79	23,516	16.8	98.5
≥80	2110	19.5	88.2

Table 1.4 The prevalence of pterygium among different ethnic groups

	Ethnic groups		
Prevalence of pterygium	Bai (%)	Yi (%)	Han (%)
Pterygium	39.00	29.50	39.50
Severe pterygium	7.50	3.80	5.20

Note: Pterygium is classified as severe when it reaches or exceeds the pupil margin

occupation, and education level) are related to the occurrence of pterygium and must be considered.

China is a multiethnic country. The prevalence of pterygium among different ethnic groups has been reported in the literature. Zhong et al. [15] conducted an epidemiological study of pterygium in various ethnic minorities living in the same rural area of Yunnan (99.58°E, 25.25°N). They found that the prevalence of pterygium was remarkably lower among the Yi ethnic population than among the Bai and Han ethnic groups and that severe pterygium was most common among Bai residents (Table 1.4).

As reported by Chen et al. [16] in an epidemiological survey of Han and Uyghur residents living in the same region of Xinjiang, the prevalence of pterygium was 11.75% overall in the region and significantly higher among Han Chinese individuals (13.18%) than Uyghur individuals (8.97%). The difference in the prevalence of pterygium may be attributable to different lifestyles between the two ethnic groups. The Uyghur people have the custom of wearing turbans or hats; therefore, UV exposure is substantially reduced, resulting in a lower prevalence of pterygium than that for Han Chinese people.

An epidemiological study conducted by Pan et al. [11] with Han and Manchu nationality residents living in Hebei province area they reported an overall prevalence of pterygium of 6.5% in the area and a statistically nonsignificant difference in the prevalence of pterygium between Han (6.2%) and Manchu Chinese (7.2%) individuals. This finding may be explained by the fact that the Manchu population living in Hebei region has a lifestyle similar to that of Han Chinese people; as a result, the prevalence of pterygium is not significantly different between two ethnic groups.

In addition, a history of smoking in a low education level, and a low household income groups are reportedly related to a higher prevalence of pterygium [17, 18]. In summary, the incidence of pterygium has multiple risk factors, which vary among geographical regions and populations.

1.1.2 Incidence

The incidence of a disease refers to the frequency of new cases of the disease in a certain population within a particular period. Determination of the incidence of a disease requires a continuous follow-up and monitoring in a certain time period; In the previous literature reference, only a small number of studies have reported the incidence of pterygium.

The Yunnan Minority Eye Study [19] included a 5-year epidemiological survey of the Bai population living in rural Yunnan (99.58°E, 25.25°N) and revealed that the overall 5-year incidence of pterygium was 6.8%, among them Bai people over 50 years old in this area. The incidence rates were higher among women (8.8%) than men (3.8%) and were 7.7% in the 50- to 59-year-old age group, 6.5% in the 60- to 69-year-old age group, and 5.6% in the >70-year-old age group.

The Beijing Eye Study [20] included a 10-year epidemiological survey of pterygium in both a rural area and an urban area in Beijing revealed that the overall 10-year incidence of pterygium was 4.9%. The incidence rates were 5.4% in 40- to 49-year-old age group, 4.7% in 50- to 59-year-old age group, 4.5% in 60- to 69-year-old age group, and 5.0% in >70-year-old age group.

1.2 Section 2: Risk Factors

1.2.1 UV Radiation

Exposure to solar UV-B radiation (UVB) is the most significant environmental factor in the development of pterygium [1]. Up to the present, research findings suggested that [21] dysfunction of limbal stem cells (LSCs) is the main cause involved in the pathogenesis of pterygium. When the light through the temporal limbus into the anterior chamber can be intensified 20-fold on the nasal limbus. Consequently, the intensified light could damage LSCs and fibroblasts at the nasal limbus, causing pterygium. Therefore, UV radiation is the main risk factor causing pterygium. People who live in rural area, participate in more outdoor activities, are employed in outdoor occupations, or live in areas with strong UV radiation are susceptible suffered pterygium.

The main source of vitamin D in human body is vitamin D production in the skin upon exposure to ultraviolet ray (UVR) irradiation, and its primary form in the body is 25-hydroxyvitamin D in serum. A Korean study objectively assessed UVB exposure by measuring serum 25-hydroxyvitamin D and then evaluated its relationship to pterygium. The study found that sunlight exposure and 25-hydroxyvitamin D were strongly associated with the occurrence of pterygium [22] (Tables 1.5 and 1.6).

Jiao et al. [10] conducted an epidemiological study of pterygium in elderly adults in rural Shandong Province. They found that the prevalence of pterygium was 10.53% overall in the region and increased with more outdoor sunlight exposure. In addition, wearing hats or sunglasses reduced the prevalence of pterygium. These results indicated that UV radiation is a risk factor for pterygium. If wearing hats and/or sunglasses during working time could prevent pterygium. The epidemiological survey from The Yunnan Minority Eye Study further revealed that outdoor occupations is only predictor of pterygium [19].

Table 1.5 Regression analysis of the association between serum 25-hydroxyvitamin D and the prevalence of pterygium

Serum 25-hydroxyvitamin D (ng mL^{-1})	Odds ratio (OR)
>30	1.565
25–30	1.545
20–25	1.8
15–20	1.535
<15	1

Table 1.6 Regression analysis of the association between sunlight exposure and the prevalence of pterygium

Length of sunlight exposure (h)	OR
>5	1.689
2–5	1.126
<2	1

1.2.2 Genetic Factors

A genetic predisposition has been implicated in the development of pterygium. Clusters of family members with pterygium have been reported in the literature. In 1987, Zhang reported a family with pterygium living in Anyue County, Sichuan Province. Pterygium occurred in 11 family members across 3 generations with a pattern of autosomal dominant inheritance [23]. A genetic analysis conducted by Hilgers et al. [24] concluded that heredity plays an important role in the high prevalence of pterygium in the region.

Recently, genetic studies of pterygium have been reported in the literature. Ozturk et al. [25] surgically obtained normal superotemporal bulbar conjunctival and pterygium specimens for *k-ras* gene sequencing from 25 patients preoperation with primary pterygium. The results showed that while the *k-ras* gene mutation did not appear in normal conjunctival tissue, missense mutations in codon 61 occurred in 7 pterygium tissue samples, including 4 cases of Glu61Arg CAA > CGA and 3 cases of Glu61Leu CAA > CTA. The difference between the 2 groups was statistically significant, suggesting that mutations in codon 61 may play an important role in the development of pterygium.

8-Hydroxydeoxyguanine (8-OHdG) is a product of oxidative damage to DNA. Human 8-hydroxyguanine DNA glycosylase 1 (hOGG1) is the main enzyme that participates in 8-OHdG repair, and a C/G polymorphism at position 1245 in exon 7 of the hOGG1 gene results in an amino acid substitution from serine (Ser) to cysteine (Cys) in codon 326.

Kau et al. [26] explored the relationship between pterygium and gene polymorphisms in a Chinese population. They found that the hOGG1 Ser326Cys polymorphism was associated with pterygium and that compared to Ser/Cys and Ser/Ser carriers, homozygous Cys/Cys carriers were more predisposed to pterygium and developed pterygium at a younger age.

However, the inheritance pattern of pterygium remains unclear. Both Mendelian and non-Mendelian inheritance in pterygium occurrence have been reported. Mendelian inheritance can be autosomal dominant, autosomal recessive, and sex chromosome linked. Non-Mendelian inheritance may be multifactorial or mitochondrial [27].

1.2.3 Correlation with Pinguecula

The view that pinguecula is the precursor of primary pterygium was first proposed by Zehender in 1869 and was supported by Fuchs, Parsons, and Alt [1]. Pinguecula refers to a pale yellow triangular raised patch resulting from degeneration of the elastic fibres in the bulbar conjunctival connective tissue on both sides of the cornea. This change in the eye is thought to be caused by long-term exposure to UV light without protection.

References

1. Foster CS, Azar DT, Dohlman CH. Smolin and Thoft's the cornea: scientific foundations and clinical practice (Chinese version translated by Li Y). Tianjin: Tianjin Science & Technology Translation & Publishing Corp.; 2007.
2. Rezvan F, Khabazkhoob M, Hooshmand E, et al. Prevalence and risk factors of pterygium: a systematic review and meta-analysis. Surv Ophthalmol. 2018;63(5):719–35.
3. Yang M, Guan Y, Kang LH, et al. Meta-analysis of prevalence of pterygium among people aged over 40 in China. Chin J Exp Ophthamol. 2019;37(3):190–6.
4. Song P, Chang X, Wang M, et al. Variations of pterygium prevalence by age, gender and geographic characteristics in China: a systematic review and meta-analysis. PLoS One. 2017;12(3):e0174587.
5. Luthra R. Frequency and risk factors for pterygium in the Barbados Eye Study. Arch Ophthalmol. 2001;119(12):1827–32.
6. Ma K, Xu L, Jie Y, et al. Prevalence of and factors associated with pterygium in adult Chinese: the Beijing Eye Study. Cornea. 2007;26(10):1184–6.
7. Wu K, He M, Xu J, et al. Pterygium in aged population in Doumen County, China. Yan Ke Xue Bao. 2002;18(3):181–4.
8. Liu L, Wu J, Geng J, et al. Geographical prevalence and risk factors for pterygium: a systematic review and meta-analysis. BMJ Open. 2013;3(11):e003787.
9. Lu P, Chen X, Kang Y, et al. Pterygium in Tibetans: a population based study in China. Clin Exp Ophthalmol. 2007;35(9):828–33.
10. Jiao WZ, Zhou CC, Wang T, et al. Prevalence and risk factors for pterygium in rural older adults in Shandong Province of China: a cross-sectional study. J Biomed Biotechnol. 2014;2014:658648.
11. Pan Z, Cui J, Shan G, et al. Prevalence and risk factors for pterygium: a cross-sectional study in Han and Manchu ethnic populations in Hebei, China. BMJ Open. 2019;9(2):e025725.
12. Yasemi M, Bamdad S, Sarokhani D, et al. Prevalence of pterygium in Iran: a systematic review and meta-analysis study. Electron Physician. 2017;9(12):5914–9.
13. Nemesure B, Wu SY, Hennis A, et al. Nine-year incidence and risk factors for pterygium in the Barbados Eye Studies. Ophthalmology. 2008;115(12):2153–8.
14. Ang M, Li X, Wong W, et al. Prevalence of and racial differences in pterygium: a multiethnic population study in Asians. Ophthalmology. 2012;119(8):1509–15.

15. Zhong H, Cha X, Wei T, et al. Prevalence of and risk factors for pterygium in rural adult Chinese populations of the Bai nationality in Dali: the Yunnan Minority Eye Study. Invest Ophthalmol Vis Sci. 2012;53(10):6617–21.
16. Chen T, Ding L, Shan G, et al. Prevalence and racial differences in pterygium: a cross-sectional study in Han and Uygur adults in Xinjiang, China. Invest Ophthalmol Vis Sci. 2015;56(2):1109–17.
17. Lin YH, Sun CC, Yeung L, et al. Epidemiologic study of pterygium in Taiwan. Jpn J Ophthalmol. 2019;63(4):297–303.
18. Saw SM, Tan D. Pterygium: prevalence, demography and risk factors. Ophthalmic Epidemiol. 1999;6(3):219–28.
19. Li L, Zhong H, Tian E, et al. Five-year incidence and predictors for pterygium in a rural community in China: the Yunnan Minority Eye Study. Cornea. 2015;34(12):1564–8.
20. Liang Z, Sheng YQ, Liang X, et al. 10-year incidence and associations of pterygium in adult Chinese: the Beijing Eye Study. Invest Opthalmol Vis Sci. 2013;54(2):1509–14.
21. Zhou W, Zhu Y, Zhang B, et al. The role of ultraviolet radiation in the pathogenesis of pterygia (Review). Mol Med Rep. 2016;14(1):3–15.
22. Chun YH, Paik JS, Oh JH, et al. Association between pterygium, sun exposure, and serum 25-hydroxyvitamin in a nationally representative sample of Korean adults. Lipids Health Dis. 2018;17(1):260.
23. Zhang JD. An investigation of aetiology and heredity of pterygium. Acta Ophthalmol. 1987;65(4):413–6.
24. Hilgers JH. Pterygium: its incidence, heredity and etiology. Am J Ophthalmol. 1960;50(4):635–44.
25. Ozturk BT, Yildirim MS, Zamani A, et al. K-ras oncogene mutation in pterygium. Eye. 2017;31(3):491–8.
26. Kau HC, Tsai CC, Hsu WM, et al. Genetic polymorphism of hOGG1 and risk of pterygium in Chinese. Eye. 2004;18(6):635–9.
27. Anguria P, Kitinya J, Ntuli S, et al. The role of heredity in pterygium development. Int J Ophthalmol. 2014;7(3):563–73.

Chapter 2
Pathogenesis and Histopathology

Shaowei Li and Kuanshu Li

2.1 Section 1: Pathogenesis

Up till now, pathogenesis of pterygium is not fully understood. Pterygium is thought to be the combined result of internal (genetic) and extrinsic (external environment) factors according to recent studies.

2.1.1 Genetic Factors

Pterygium has a genetic predisposition. Studies have reported clusters of family members with pterygium. Zhang [1] reported a family with pterygium living in Anyue County, Sichuan Province, in China. Eleven family members across three generations had pterygium, suggesting an autosomal dominant inheritance pattern [1].

P53 is a major tumor suppressor that plays a pivotal role in maintaining gene stability and regulating the cell cycle, apoptosis, differentiation, and DNA repair. In the immunohistochemical tests conducted by Weinstein et al., p53 overexpression in pterygium tissue was present in 7 of 13 patients, suggesting that pterygium may result from uncontrolled cell proliferation. Tan et al. [2] also revealed abnormal expression of p53 in the epithelial tissue of both primary and recurrent pterygium.

Previous studies [3, 4] have found that the environmental pollutant benzo[a]pyrene (BaP), a polycyclic aromatic hydrocarbon (PAH), can cause p53 mutations. BaP

S. Li (✉)
Beijing Aier Intech Eye Hospital, Beijing, China
e-mail: lishaowei@aierchina.com

K. Li
Changsha Aier Eye Hospital, Changsha, China

C. Wang, S. Li (eds.), *Pterygium Surgery*,
https://doi.org/10.1007/978-981-99-6843-5_2

7,8-diol-9,10-epoxide (BPDE), which is an ultimate metabolite of BaP, attacks deoxyguanosine to form a BPDE-N2-dG adduct that results in p53 mutations. Currently, DNA adducts induced by BaP and other PAHs are used as biomarkers of p53 mutations. Tung et al. [5] reported that BPDE-like DNA adducts were found in 33% of pterygium specimens and that BPDE-like DNA adduct levels were related to *CYP1A1* gene polymorphisms. The BPDE-like DNA adduct level in patients with the *CYP1A1 m1/m2* (C/T) and *m2/m2* (T/T) genotypes was 9.675-fold higher than that in patients with the *CYP1A1 m1/m1* (C/C) genotype, indicating that the development of pterygium is associated with gene polymorphisms.

In addition, pterygium is reportedly related to *k-ras* mutations [6] and *hOGG1 Ser326Cys* polymorphisms [7]. However, the inheritance pattern of pterygium has not yet been fully identified and requires further study.

2.1.2 The Role of UV Irradiation

The solar light that causes pterygium might be in the spectral wavelength range between 280 and 315 nm, known as UVB light. Cellular DNA is known to readily absorb UV light at a wavelength of 260 nm. UV light coming from the temporal side and refracted by the temporal cornea passes through the anterior chamber and focuses on the nasal limbus; consequently, the UV light energy highly concentrated on the nasal limbus leads to photobiological reactions that target DNA molecules.

Existing research on the relationship between UV radiation and pterygium mainly focuses on the following aspects:

1. **Damage to limbal stem cells (LSCs)** Light irradiation of the temporal limbus can be focused and intensified 20 times at the nasal limbus after it passes through the anterior chamber, potentially damaging the LSCs and fibroblasts at the nasal limbus and resulting in the occurrence of pterygium [8].
2. **Oxidative stress** Exposure to UV radiation can produce massive reactive oxygen radicals in tissue, i.e., oxidative stress, which can damage DNA and proteins in cells. The expression of 8-hydroxydeoxyguanosine (8-OHDG), a sensitive biomarker of DNA oxidative damage, is excessively high in pterygium tissue but relatively low in normal conjunctival tissue [9]. Mehmet et al. [10] revealed that the enzyme activities of catalase (CAT), superoxide dismutase (SOD), and glutathione peroxidase (GSH-Px) were significantly lower and the levels of nitric oxide (NO) and malondialdehyde (MDA) were significantly higher in pterygium tissue than in normal conjunctival tissue. These findings indicate that oxidative stress plays an important role in the formation of pterygium.
3. **Activation of signaling pathways** Sphingosine 1 phosphate (S1P) is a bioactive lipid that regulates cell activity and has important functions such as regulating cellular proliferation, migration, and fibrosis. UV radiation activates the S1P-RhoA signaling pathway and upregulates the expression of S1P, and pterygium tissue has been found to have a significantly higher level of S1P than normal

conjunctival tissue [11]. Urokinase plasminogen activator (uPA) is a serine that degrades the extracellular matrix (ECM), stimulates cell migration, proliferation, and chemotaxis, inhibits apoptosis, and induces angiogenesis. Chao et al. [12] found that uPA expression was significantly elevated in pterygium tissue and that UVA irradiation upregulated uPA expression through the ERK and JNK signaling pathways. These findings indicate that UV irradiation contributes to the formation of pterygium by activating signaling pathways.

4. **Induced cytokine production** UVB can induce the production of a variety of cytokines and growth factors, including interleukin (IL)-1, IL-8, tumor necrosis factor (TNF)-B, fibroblast growth factor (FGF)-2, vascular endothelial growth factor (VEGF), heparin-bound EGF (HB-EGF), transforming growth factor (TGF)-C, and stem cell factor (SCF). These factors are overexpressed in pterygium tissue and play an important role in various biological processes, such as angiogenesis and cell proliferation [13]. Therefore, the UVB-induced production of cytokines and growth factors may be involved in the pathogenesis of pterygium.

2.1.3 The Theory of LSC Limbal Barrier Disruption

LSCs serve as the metabolic and regenerative source of corneal epithelial cells. Normal LSCs form a barrier to prevent conjunctival tissue from growing into the cornea; that is, hypertrophic conjunctival fibroblasts and new blood vessels may grow onto the surface of the cornea if this barrier is disrupted. LSCs are located in the basal layer of the limbal epithelium, where LSCs can be damaged by long-term UV irradiation (the "Coroneo" effect) [14].

2.1.4 The Theory of Abnormal Cell Proliferation and Apoptosis

Pterygium is considered a hyperplasia-related disease because a large number of proliferative blood vessels and fibroblast-derived elastic and collagen fibers can be found in pterygium tissue. Liang et al. [15] found that the expression levels of the cell proliferation-related factors proliferating cell nuclear antigen (PCNA) and K-67 and the apoptosis-related factors Bcl-2 and mP53 were significantly higher in pterygium tissue than in normal conjunctival tissue. Mammalian target of rapamycin (mTOR) is an important autophagy inhibitor and regulator of cell metabolism. mTOR, especially mTORC1, is highly activated in pterygium tissue, and mTORC1 stimulates cell proliferation by negatively modulating fibroblast growth factor receptor 3 (FGFR3) and inhibits apoptosis by inhibiting the expression of the autophagy factor LC3 and the apoptotic factor bcl-2 [16]. These findings suggest that abnormal cell hyperplasia and apoptosis may play important roles in the occurrence of pterygium.

2.1.5 The Cytokine Theory

Pterygium tissue contains a large number of inflammatory factors, growth factors, and growth factor receptors, which are related to damage caused by UVB exposure. Existing studies have mainly focused on the cytokines listed below.

1. **ILs** IL-1, IL-6, and IL-8 are the main cytokines involved in pterygium. Di Girolamo et al. [17] found that UVB induced IL-6 and IL-8 production; the abundant expression of these two ILs in pterygium epithelial cells promoted angiogenesis, cell proliferation, tissue invasion, and the inflammatory response, thus playing a crucial role in the formation of pterygium.
2. **TNF** Kria et al. [18] revealed that TNF-α is expressed in the epithelial and stromal cells of pterygium and that UVB or IL-1 induces TNF-α production, which mediates the release of various inflammatory factors and chemokines to induce neovascularization.
3. **VEGF** UVB can upregulate VEGF expression [19]. High VEGF expression is present in pterygium tissue, suggesting that VEGF may be involved in the proliferation and neovascularization of pterygium [20, 21].
4. **Epidermal growth factor receptor (EGFR)** The EGFR family includes a class of receptors associated with proliferation, e.g., EGFR, ErbB-2, ErbB-3, and ErbB-4. Research [22] has shown that EGFR, ErbB-2, and ErbB-3 are expressed only in superficial cells in normal conjunctival tissue but are overexpressed in all pterygium tissue layers, indicating that pterygium is a proliferative disease.
5. **Basic fibroblast growth factor (b-FGF)** b-FGF strongly promotes neovascularization. It is strongly expressed in pterygium epithelial cells, stromal fibroblasts, and vascular endothelial cells [18] and is even more significantly expressed in cultured fibroblasts of recurrent pterygium [23]. UVB can upregulate b-FGF expression [24]. These findings suggest that b-FGF may be involved in the formation and development of pterygium.

Additionally, HB-EGF [25], TGF-β [18], and platelet-derived growth factor (PDGF) [18], which play important roles in various biological processes, including angiogenesis and cell proliferation, have been detected in pterygium tissue. Activation of these factors may be related to the occurrence of pterygium.

2.1.6 The Extracellular Matrix Remodeling Theory

Pterygium can lead to remodeling of the ECM, including degeneration of elastic fibers and deterioration of anterior corneal elasticity, processes in which matrix metalloproteinases (MMPs) play an important role. MMPs belong to a complex protease family that depends on catalytic zinc ions for its action and hydrolyses the components of the ECM as substrates to participate in the destruction and remodeling of the ECM. MMP-1 and MMP-3 levels were found to be higher in pterygium head fibroblasts than in pterygium body, subconjunctival, and normal conjunctival fibroblasts, suggesting that ECM remodeling may be responsible for the growth and corneal invasion of pterygium [26].

2.2 Section 2: Histopathology

Primary pterygium is anatomically divided into three parts: the head, neck, and body. The pterygium head is located on the corneal surface, the neck is located at the limbus, and the body is located above the sclera. The main histopathological changes in pterygium include the following:

1. Epithelial changes similar to conjunctival epithelium atrophy. Conjunctival epithelial cells cross the limbus and cover the thickened, hypertrophic, and degenerated connective tissue of the pterygium.
2. Abnormal proliferation of subepithelial fibroblasts. Degeneration of elastic fibers in pterygium is characterized by the aggregation of abnormal collagen tissues into vortex-like and fibrous shapes, which are basophilic and appear similar to elastic tissue. A large number of neovascular blood vessels are scattered between the coarse collagen fibers, which provide blood supply to the degenerated tissue.
3. Fusion of the pterygium body and Tenon's capsule underneath. Such fusion does not affect the superficial scleral tissue. Therefore, clinically, most pterygium cases show good mobility and without adherence to the sclera.
4. Adhesion between the pterygium neck and limbus. Due to the absence of Tenon's capsule, the pterygium neck tightly adheres to the superficial tissue of the sclera underneath at the limbus. The adhesion is so strong that a surgical probe cannot easily pass through and the tissues are difficult to separate during surgery. This is one of the key criteria for differentiating primary pterygium from pseudopterygium [27].
5. Location of the pterygium head between the Bowmen layer and epithelial basement membrane (EBM) of the cornea. The pterygium head invades the area between the Bowmen layer and EBM. A row of fibroblasts is present in the anterior pterygium head, along which the pterygium head invades the corneal tissue. During this invasive process, the Bowman layer is pushed backward by fibroblasts and ultimately ruptures, allowing fibrovascular tissue to grow into the superficial layer of the corneal stroma, forming a firm bond between the pterygium head and the corneal tissue [27].
6. Pterygium is pathologically composed of degenerated subepithelial fibrous tissue that is basophilic and strongly positive on elastic fiber staining. Hogan and Alvarado [28] found that only a portion of fibers in pterygium are sensitive to elastase and therefore speculated that collagen fiber degeneration might be the reason for the resistance to elastase.

7. The relationship between pterygium morphology and histopathology. Safi et al. [29] revealed that in pterygium, the degree of congestion (redness) was related solely to vascular density and not to other histopathological factors. Fleshiness was related only to stromal fibrosis, and the dimensions of the pterygium lesion passing the corneal limbus were related to vascular density but not stromal elastosis.
8. No significant differences identified between primary and recurrent pterygium histopathology. Nuhoglu et al. [30] compared 90 eyes of 90 patients with primary pterygium and 11 eyes of 11 patients with recurrent pterygium. They found no significant difference in inflammation intensity, the degree of vascularization, or fibrinoid degeneration between primary and recurrent pterygium. Of the 90 patients who had primary pterygium, no significant histopathological difference was found between patients with (7/90) and without recurrence (83/90). Of the 11 patients with recurrent pterygium, no histopathological difference was detected between patients with (2/11) and without recurrence (9/11), suggesting no significant associations between histopathological characteristics and pterygium recurrence.

References

1. Zhang JD. An investigation of aetiology and heredity of pterygium. Acta Ophthalmol. 1987;65(4):413–6.
2. Tan DT, Lim AS, Goh HS, et al. Abnormal expression of the p53 tumor suppressor gene in the conjunctiva of patients with pterygium. Am J Ophthalmol. 1997;123(3):404–5.
3. Kuo CY, Cheng YW, Chen CY, et al. Correlation between the amounts of polycyclic aromatic hydrocarbons and mutagenicity of airborne particulate samples from Taichung City, Taiwan. Environ Res. 1998;78(1):43–9.
4. Hussain SP, Amstad P, Raja K, et al. Mutability of p53 hotspot codons to benzo(a)pyrene diol epoxide (BPDE) and the frequency of p53 mutations in nontumorous human lung. Cancer Res. 2001;61(17):6350–5.
5. Tung JN, Wu HH, Chiang CC, et al. An association between BPDE-like DNA adduct levels and CYP1A1 and GSTM1 polymorphisma in pterygium. Mol Vis. 2010;16:623–9.
6. Ozturk BT, Yildirim MS, Zamani A, et al. Kras oncogene mutation in pterygium. Eye. 2017;31(3):491–8.
7. Kau HC, Tsai CC, Hsu WM, et al. Genetic polymorphism of hOGG1 and risk of pterygium in Chinese. Eye. 2004;18(6):635–9.
8. Zhou W, Zhu Y, Zhang B, et al. The role of ultraviolet radiation in the pathogenesis of pterygia (Review). Mol Med Rep. 2016;14(1):3–15.
9. Perra MT, Maxia C, Corbu A, et al. Oxidative stress in pterygium: relationship between p53 and 8-hydroxydeoxyguanosine. Mol Vis. 2006;12:1136–42.
10. Mehmet B, Semsettin S, Fatih MM, et al. Investigation of oxidative stress in pterygium tissue. Mol Vis. 2011;17:443–7.
11. Nozomi I, Megumi H, Takashi F, et al. Activation of the sphingosine 1 Phosphate-Rho pathway in pterygium and in ultraviolet-irradiated normal conjunctiva. Int J Mol Sci. 2019;20(19):4670.
12. Chao SC, Hu DN, Yang PY, et al. Ultraviolet-A irradiation upregulated urokinase-type plasminogen activator in pterygium fibroblasts through ERK and JNK pathways. Invest Ophthalmol Vis Sci. 2013;54(2):999–1007.

13. Chui J, Girolamo ND, Wakefield D, et al. The pathogenesis of pterygium: current concepts and their therapeutic implications. Ocul Surf. 2008;6(1):24–43.
14. Coroneo MT, Di Girolamo N, Wakefield D. The pathogenesis of pterygia. Curr Opin Opthalmol. 1999;10(4):282–8.
15. Liang K, Jiang Z, Ding BQ, et al. Expression of cell proliferation and apoptosis biomarkers in pterygia and normal conjunctiva. Mol Vis. 2011;17:1687–93.
16. Liu Y, Xu H, An M. mTORC1 regulates apoptosis and cell proliferation in pterygium by targeting autophagy and FGFR3. Sci Rep. 2017;7:7339.
17. Di Girolamo N, Kumar RK, Coroneo MT, et al. UVB-mediated induction of interleukin-6 and -8 in pterygia and cultured human pterygium epithelial cells. Invest Ophthalmol Vis Sci. 2002;43(11):3430–7.
18. Kria L, Ohira A, Amemiya T. Immunohistochemical localization of basic fibroblast growth factor, platelet derived growth factor, transforming growth factor and tumor necrosis factor in the pterygium. Acta Histochem. 1996;98(2):195–201.
19. Blaudschun R, Sunderkötter C, Brenneisen P, et al. Vascular endothelial growth factor causally contributes to the angiogenic response upon ultraviolet B irradiation. Br J Dermatol. 2002;146(4):581–7.
20. Lee DH, Cho HJ, Kim JT, et al. Expression of vascular endothelial growth factor and inducible nitric oxide synthase in pterygia. Cornea. 2001;20(7):738–42.
21. Marcovich AL, Morad Y, Sandbank J, et al. Angiogenesis in pterygium: morphometric and immunohistochemical study. Curr Eye Res. 2009;25(1):17–22.
22. Liu Z, Xie Y, Zhang M. Overexpression of type I growth factor receptors in pterygium. Chin Med J. 2002;115(3):418–21.
23. Kria L, Ohira A, Amemiya T. Growth factors in cultured pterygium fibroblasts: immunohistochemical and ELISA analysis. Graefes Arch Clin Exp Ophthalmol. 1998;236(9):702–8.
24. Ley RD, Miska KB, Kusewitt DF. Photoreactivation of ultraviolet radiation induced basic fibroblast growth factor (bFGF) and the role of bFGF in corneal lesion formation in Monodelphis domestica. Environ Mol Mutagen. 2001;38(23):175–9.
25. Nolan TM, Digirolamo N, Sachdev NH, et al. The role of ultraviolet irradiation and heparin-binding epidermal growth factor-like growth factor in the pathogenesis of pterygium. Am J Pathol. 2003;162(2):567–74.
26. Li DQ, Lee SB, Gunja-Smith Z, et al. Overexpression of collagenase (MMP1) and stromelysin (MMP3) by pterygium head fibroblasts. Arch Ophthalmol. 2001;119(1):71–80.
27. Foster CS, Azar DT, Dohlman CH. Smolin and Thoft's the cornea: scientific foundations and clinical practice (Chinese version translated by Li Y). Tianjin: Tianjin Science & Technology Translation & Publishing Corp.; 2007.
28. Hogan MJ, Alvarado J. Pterygium and pinguecula: electron microscopic study. Arch Ophthalmol. 1967;78(2):174–86.
29. Safi H, Kheirkhah A, Mahbod M, et al. Correlations between histopathologic changes and clinical features in pterygia. J Ophthalmic Vis Res. 2016;11(2):153–8.
30. Nuhoglu F, Turna F, Uyar M, et al. Is there a relation between histopathologic characteristics of pterygium and recurrence rates? Eur J Ophthalmol. 2013;23(3):303–8.

Part II
Clinical Practice

Chapter 3
Clinical Features, Diagnosis, and Treatment of Pterygium

Congxiang Wang

Pterygium is clinically divided into three categories based on pathogenesis and etiology:

- Primary pterygium (also called real pterygium)
- Recurrent pterygium
- Pseudo pterygium

The etiology of primary pterygium remains unclear. Most scholars considered that the occurrence of primary pterygium is associated with UV exposure in most cases and genetic factors in some cases. Recurrent pterygium is defined as the regrowth of primary pterygium into the corneal limbus after extraction surgery. Pseudopterygium, which is not primary pterygium, results from conjunctival trauma, inflammation, or autoimmune disease complications.

3.1 Section 1: Clinical Manifestations and Diagnosis of Primary Pterygium

3.1.1 Symptoms

1. **Foreign body sensation** Patients with pterygium often have a gritty feeling in the eyes, as the symptom of dry eye. Due to excessive exposure to UV light, wind, and environment, overgrowth of pterygium into the surface of the cornea and elevated above the bulbar conjunctiva leads to interfere and/or obstruct the lacrimal fluid flow and meibomian gland dysfunction (MGD) in patients with pterygium. Pterygium overgrowth into the corneal surface could cause dynamic

C. Wang (✉)
Changsha Aier Eye Hospital, Changsha, China

C. Wang, S. Li (eds.), *Pterygium Surgery*,
https://doi.org/10.1007/978-981-99-6843-5_3

abnormality in tear flow (Fig. 3.1a). Severe MGD can cause lipid abnormalities in the tear film; the patient in Fig. 3.1b had dry eye symptoms resulting from mixed causes, i.e., lipid abnormalities on the surface of cornea and tear fluid kinetic abnormalities from dry eye.

2. **Dry and itchy sensation** Patients with primary pterygium have significant dry eye symptoms. In addition to the cause of dry eye mentioned above, *Demodex* mites in eyelash hair follicles are responsible for dry and itchy eye symptoms in some patients. *Demodex* mites in eyelash hair follicles is one of the causes of pterygium recurrence after surgery (Fig. 3.2).

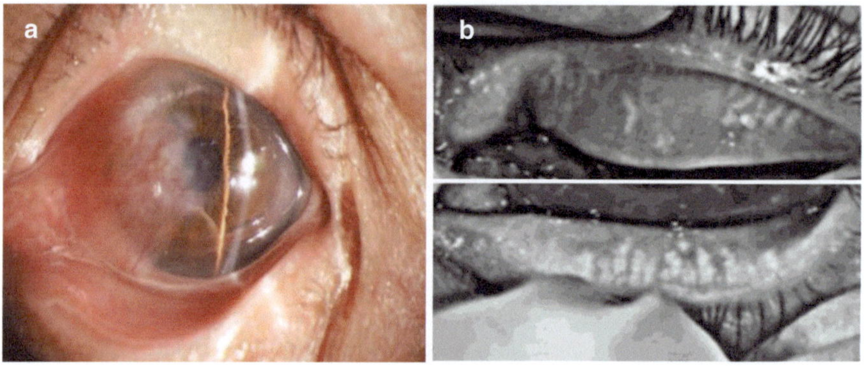

Fig. 3.1 Pterygium with MGD. (**a**) Pterygium protruding from the conjunctival surface to the cornea affects the tear fluid drainage, causing abnormal tear fluid drainage and an orifice obstruction of all upper and lower meibomian glands at the posterior eyelid margin. (**b**) Meibomian gland imaging shows a loss of more than 2/3 of the meibomian glands, i.e., severe MGD

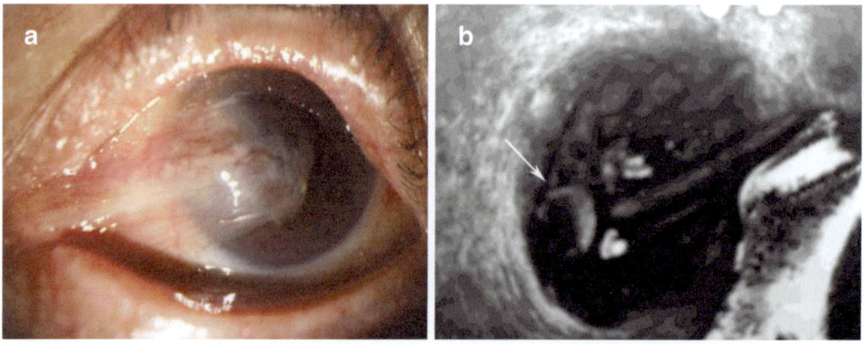

Fig. 3.2 Pterygium complicated with *Demodex* mites in eyelash hair follicles. (**a**) In addition to mixed dry eye, scaly secretions are present at the roots of the eyelash hair at the anterior margin of the upper eyelid; obstruction of the orifice occurs in more than 2/3 of the upper and lower meibomian glands at the posterior eyelid margin; lipid caps and plugs, as well as lipid opacification in eye lid, are present in the orifices of a small number of meibomian glands that remain open. (**b**) Laser confocal microscopy shows a large number of *Demodex* mites in the eyelash hair follicles (white arrow)

3. **Eye redness and limited eyeball movement** In patients with active stage of pterygium, redness of the eye results from a noninfectious inflammatory response of corneal and conjunctival epithelial cells and noninfectious inflammation in the bulbar conjunctiva caused by the pterygium lesion. Some patients have restricted eyeball movement towards the opposite side of the pterygium because large pterygium pulls on the lacrimal caruncle and causes symblepharon (Fig. 3.3).

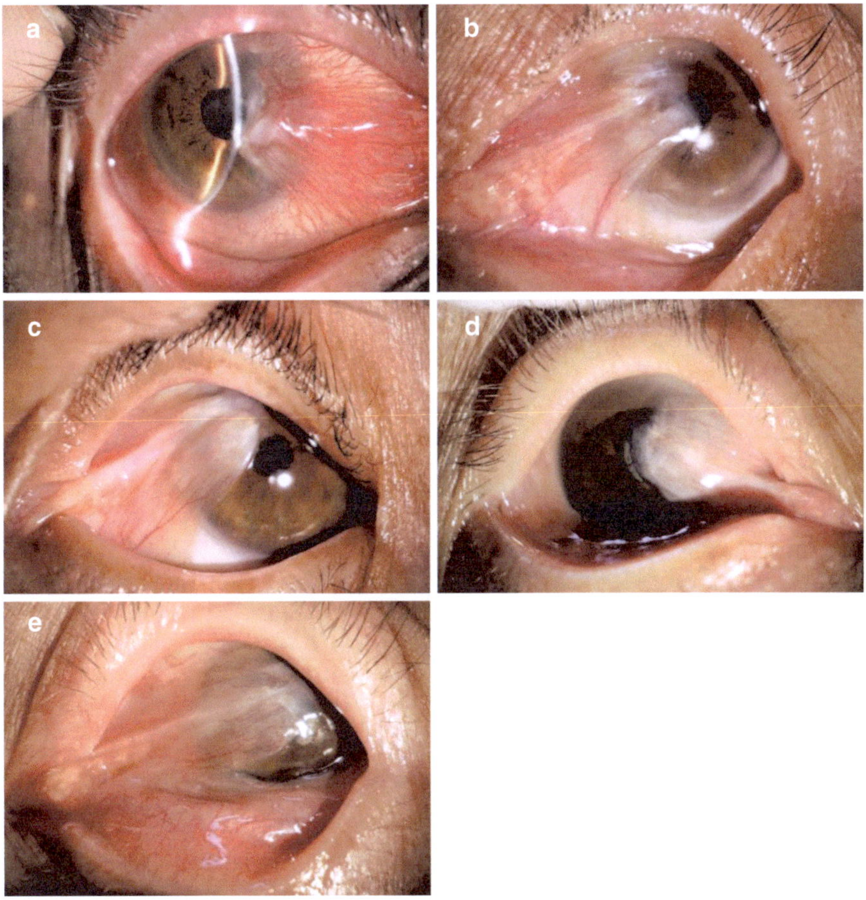

Fig. 3.3 Eye redness and limited eyeball mobility are present in a portion of patients with primary pterygium. (**a**) Active pterygium: in patients with active pterygium, conjunctival congestion and noninfectious inflammation may occur and must be controlled prior to the surgical treatment of pterygium. (**b**) Symblepharon: some patients have a limited ability to roll the eyeball towards the temporal side due to conjunctival adherence to the cornea at the lacrimal caruncle. (**c**) Conjunctival adherence at the lacrimal caruncle to the cornea above in a patient with primary pterygium. (**d**) In a patient with primary pterygium, conjunctival adherence at the lacrimal caruncle to the cornea limits the ability of the eyeball to roll towards the temporal side. (**e**) In a patient with primary pterygium, conjunctival adherence at the lacrimal caruncle to the cornea limits the mobility of the eyeball

4. **Vision acuity decreased** Invasion of pterygium into the cornea could flatten the horizontal meridian of the cornea and result in corneal astigmatism, which manifests as blurred or decreased visual acuity; large pterygium can cause up to 1.5 D with-the-rule astigmatism of the cornea [1]. In patients whose pterygium does not cover the pupil, astigmatism can be treated with refractive correction. In patients with declined vision due to pterygium close to or even covering the pupil, vision might not significantly improve with refractive correction (Fig. 3.4).
5. **Photophobia and lacrimation** Dry eye is one of the essential cause of photophobia and lacrimation. In addition to MGD and kinetic abnormalities in tears outflow, the obstruction or narrowing of the lacrimal duct system may contribute

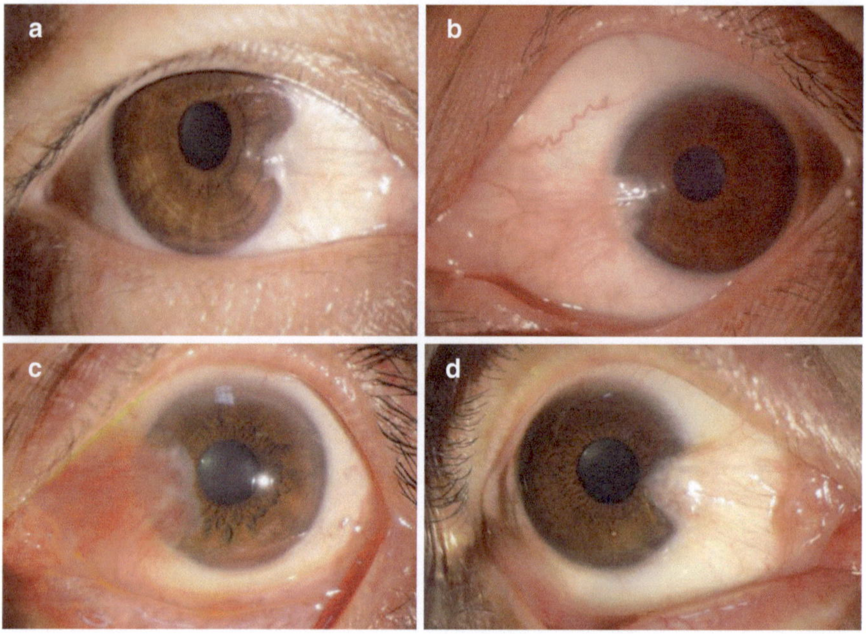

Fig. 3.4 Impact of different pterygium sizes on visual acuity. (**a**) Small pterygium is little impact on the patient's vision. The patient had an uncorrected visual acuity of 1.2 with mild astigmatism. Pterygium did not cause any symptoms, and correction for astigmatism was unnecessary. (**b**) Smaller pterygium little impact on the patient's vision. The patient with family history of pterygium had visual acuity of 1.0 without correction with a mild astigmatism. Pterygium surgery was requested to improve his looks. The patient was 32 years old and had a family history of pterygium; therefore, the risk of postoperative recurrence was high, and the surgery should be performed by a senior physician who had extensive experience in pterygium surgery. (**c**) Pterygium extending and close to the pupil may have affected the patient's visual acuity. The patient had an uncorrected vision of 0.8, with-the-rule astigmatism of 1.25 D, and best-corrected vision was 1.2. (**d**) Pterygium extending or close to the pupil may have affected the patient's vision. The patient had an uncorrected vision of 0.8, astigmatism of 1.5 D, and best-corrected vision acuity was 1.5. (**e–f**) Giant pterygium covered the pupil, causing blindness in the patient; pre-operation the patient's visual acuity was "hand movement (HM) ". (**g**) Giant pterygium covered the pupil, causing blindness in a patient; the patient's visual acuity was "counting fingers (CF)" in front of the eye

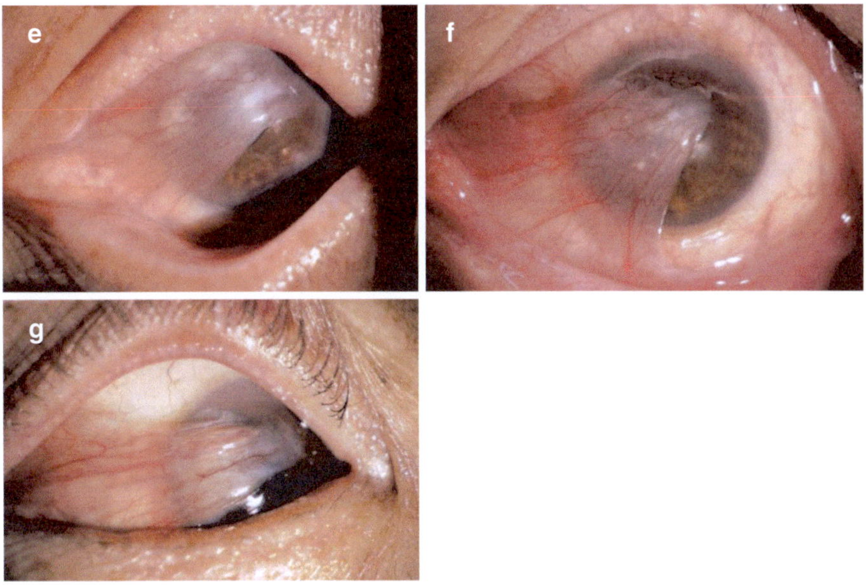

Fig. 3.4 (continued)

to lacrimation in patients with primary pterygium, by lacrimal duct irrigation to determine the existence of a lacrimal drainage duct system problem. Further more dry eye could associate with MGD-caused lipid abnormalities, it is necessary to fully communicate with patients before surgery and understand postoperative treatment and medication; such treatment could help alleviate dry eye symptoms after surgery and make them comfortably use their eyes.

6. **Cosmetic problems Patients** even with a small pterygium can affect cosmetic appearance, and moderate and severe pterygium can affect the appearance of the eye more prominently (Fig. 3.5).

3.1.2 Signs

1. **Corneal astigmatism** Primary pterygium that has invaded into the corneal limbus more than 3 mm can flatten the corneal horizontal meridian and cause relatively severe with-the-rule astigmatism of the cornea. In patients with both cataracts and pterygium, pre-operation is difficult to ensure the accuracy of intraocular lens calculations due to corneal astigmatism; hence, pterygium surgery should be performed prior to cataract surgery (Figs. 4.9 and 4.10).
2. **Congestion** Active pterygium often causes significant congestion and white filamentous discharge of the bulbar conjunctiva in the lesioned area (Fig. 3.6).
3. **Growth of membranous-like neoplastic tissue from the conjunctiva into the corneal limbus** Primary pterygium usually occurs in the nasal or temporal inter-

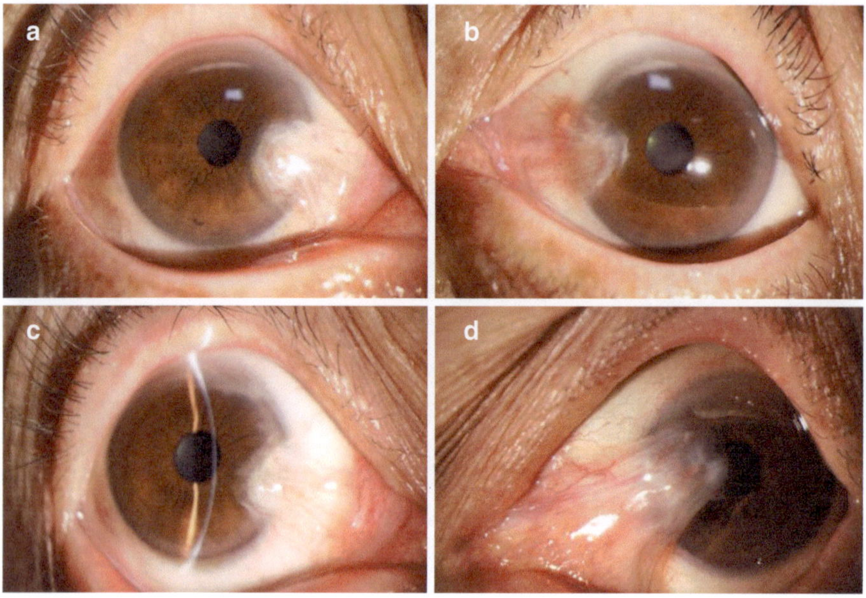

Fig. 3.5 Cosmetic disturbance caused by pterygium. (**a**, **b**) A 42-year-old patient had pterygium in both eyes and reported serious and negative effects on her cosmetic appearance, employment and marriage. (**c**) A 51-year-old patient asked for surgical treatment to improve his cosmetic appearance because pterygium affected his ability to find a job. (**d**) A 61-year-old patient asked for surgical treatment because the negative effects on her cosmetic appearance affected her plan of going to visit Shanghai with her son

palpebral fissure area. It grows horizontally towards the central pupil area or superior/inferior to the pupil area [2]. Corneal stromal degeneration may occur in the long-term pterygium, its head attached area, and conjunctival cysts may also occur on its head, neck, or body of a small number of primary pterygium (Figs. 3.10 and 3.16).

3.1.3 Growth and Characteristics of Pterygium During Different Stages

Primary pterygium presents as a triangular fleshy growth and looks as a "bird wing" shape. Primary pterygium is usually anatomically divided into three parts: head, neck, and body (Fig. 3.7). The pterygium head, which is located on the corneal surface, invasively grows between the corneal Bowmen layer and EBM. The pterygium neck, which is located at the corneal limbus, often adheres directly to the superficial sclera because there is no Tenon's capsule underneath. The pterygium body fuses with Tenon's capsule underneath without invading the superficial sclera [1].

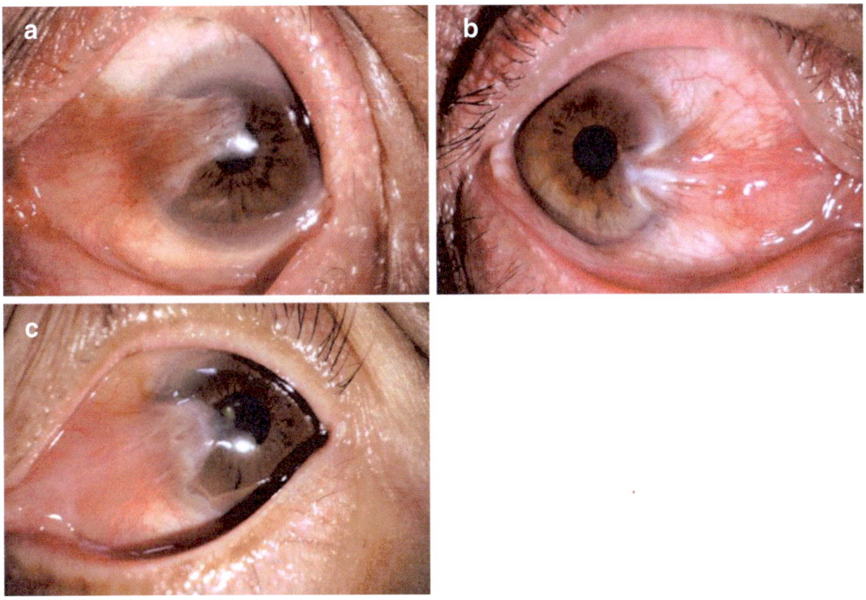

Fig. 3.6 Varying degrees of local conjunctival congestion caused by primary pterygium. (**a**) Primary pterygium-caused congestion manifested as eye redness and lacrimation, which increased deteriorate via wind exposure; (**b**) primary pterygium-caused congestion manifested as eye redness and lacrimation, which deteriorated via wind exposure; (**c**) primary pterygium-caused congestion manifested as redness and lacrimation of the eye

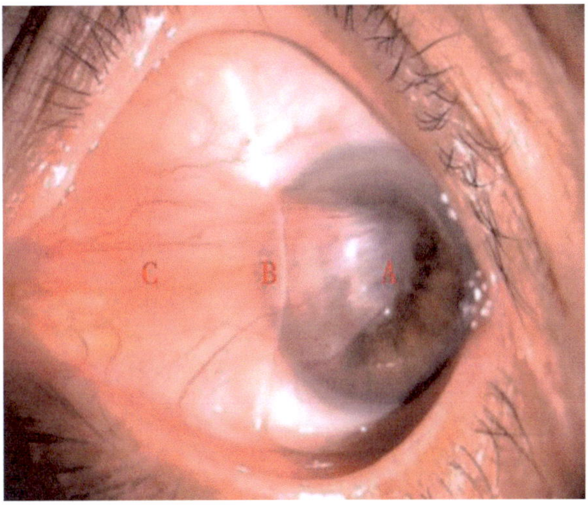

Fig. 3.7 Subdivision of the pterygium. Pterygium areas. Area A is the head part of the pterygium: the part between the Bowman layer and the epithelial basement membrane; Area B is the neck part of the pterygium: the part of the pterygium in the corneal limbus, which tightly adheres to the corneal limbus due to the absence of Tenon's cyst below, and the probe cannot pass through; Area C is the body part of the pterygium: the part above the sclera, which tightly integrates with the Tenon's cyst, but does not invade the sclera, and it is easily detached from the scleral surface during surgery

Partial head tip of the pterygium reached the margin of the pupil and superficial greyish-white small island infiltration with calcification can be surgically removed completely (Fig. 3.8). For pterygium with a visible dark-brown iron deposition line (Stocker's line) in the Bowmen layer at the tip of its head, which is caused by iron sedimentation in the tear pool formed by the corneal leading edge of the pterygium [1], should be careful peeling and separating during surgery (Fig. 3.9).

In some patients with a long-standing pterygium or excessively wide arcus senilis (corneal arcus), it is impossible to remove the degenerative lesions in the deep corneal stroma that are connected to arcus senilis at the attachment site of the pterygium head and local degenerative deep stromal lesions at the pterygium attachment site completely by surgery. This situation needs to talk and explained to patients and their relatives before surgery (Fig. 3.10).

3.1.3.1 Growth Characteristics of Pterygium

1. **General characteristics of growth** Primary pterygium mostly grows along or around the nasal horizonal line unilaterally, but bilateral involvement can also occur. Nasal pterygium is the most common type of pterygium, accounting for 60% of cases (Fig. 3.7), and temporal pterygium accounts for approximately 20% of cases (Fig. 3.11). "Double pterygium" refers to pterygium growth on

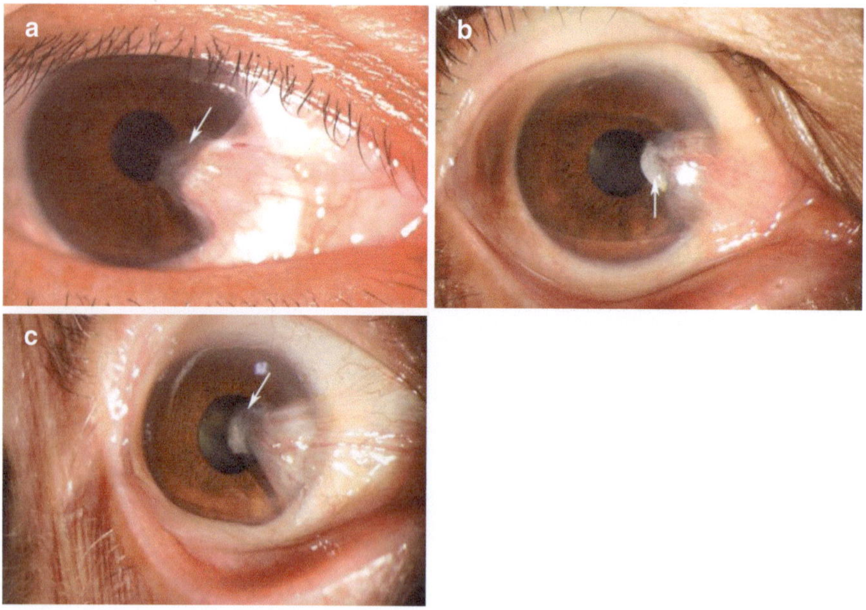

Fig. 3.8 (**a–c**) Gray small island-like infiltration on the head of pterygium (indicated by white arrow), which is indicated the invasion of the head of the pterygium involved the cornea and the fusion with the basement membrane of the cornea

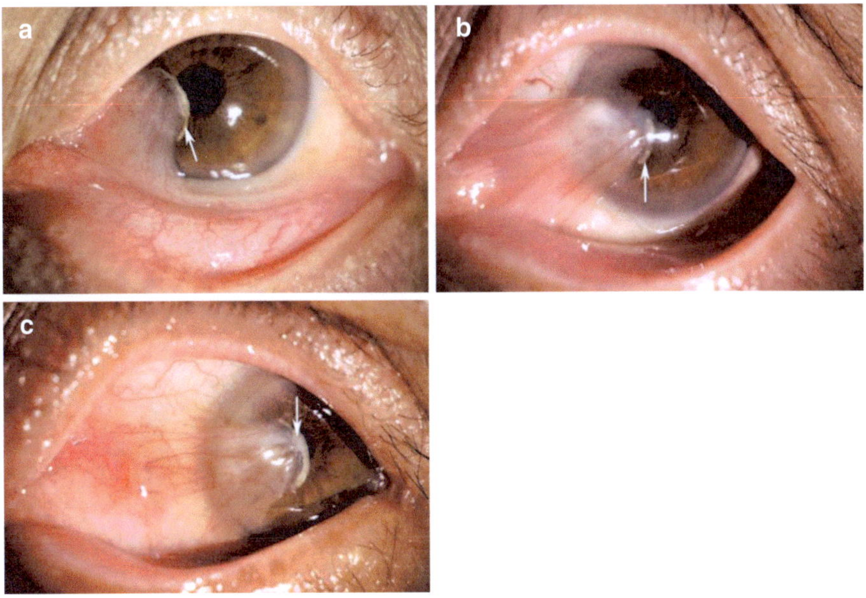

Fig. 3.9 (**a–c**) Stocker line: iron deposit formed from the tear pool at the anterior edge of the cornea on the head part of the pterygium (indicated by white arrow), it is commonly seen in elderly patients, pterygium with Stocker line is often in the quiescent phase, peeling with patience is required during surgery

both the nasal and temporal sides of the same eye (Fig. 3.12); "bilateral pterygium" and "bilateral double pterygium" refer to pterygium growth on one side of both eyes [1] (Fig. 3.13) or both sides of both eyes (Fig. 3.14), respectively. Pterygium with two or more heads is called "double-headed pterygium" or "multi-headed pterygium" (Fig. 3.15).

In a small number of primary pterygia that have tubular glands aligned parallel to epithelial cells and large empty spaces between tissues, conjunctival cysts may form (Fig. 3.16). The cyst membrane removed during surgery should be pathologically examined; most cysts are benign.

2. **Characteristics of horizontal growth pterygium** This type of primary pterygium grows along the epithelium and does not invade the stroma of the cornea. Hence, the pterygium head can be lifted to allow complete separation of the pterygium from the cornea during surgery. The corneal wound surface is often even and smooth after pterygium removal, and the patient has only minor corneal astigmatism after surgical treatment. This type of surgery can be performed by a beginner surgeon (Fig. 3.17).

   Horizontal pterygium has the following characteristics: small islands of calcification often present on the tip of the pterygium; being at the stationary phase most of the cases; more common among seen in older patients with a long history and appearance as growth underneath the corneal epithelium.

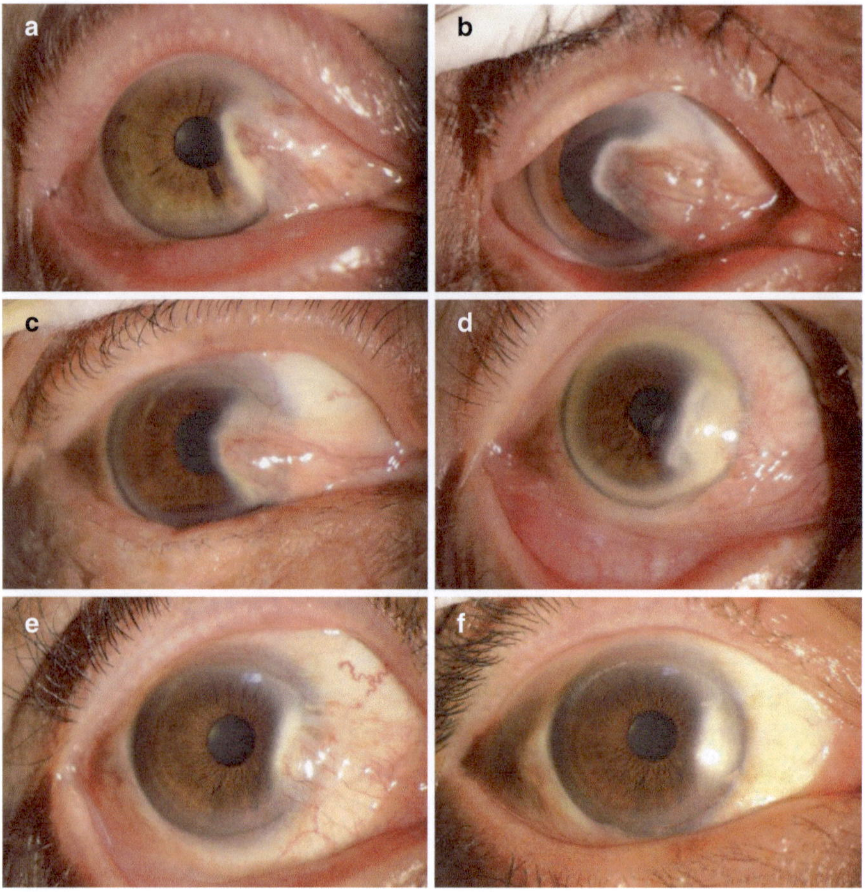

Fig. 3.10 Stromal degeneration and opacity of the cornea underneath the pterygium at its attachment site. (**a**) A degenerative lesion on the deep corneal stroma at the pterygium attachment site cannot be excised surgically, and the patient's vision might remain affected after surgery if the lesion is located in the central cornea. This situation should be talked and explained to the patients and their relatives before surgery. (**b**) A degenerative lesion on the corneal stroma at the pterygium located at the pupil area and cannot be excised by conventional pterygium surgery; as a result, the patient's vision might be reduced by plague on the cornea after surgery. This situation should be explained to the patient and the family members during the preoperative assessment. (**c**) Degenerative lesions on the corneal stroma were observed at the pterygium attachment site, and a degenerative corneal lesion could not be surgically removed. (**d**) A degenerative lesion on the corneal stroma at the pterygium attachment site is connected to the arcus senilis and cannot be excised surgically. (**e**) A degenerative lesion on the corneal stroma at the pterygium attachment site may not be able to be excised along with the pterygium during surgery; this situation should be explained to and understood by the patient and the family members. (**f**) A patient showed in (**e**) understood that the degenerative stromal lesion remained after pterygium surgery and was very satisfied with the surgical outcome. (**g**) Plaque caused by stromal degeneration remained on the cornea after surgery for primary pterygium. This situation must be clearly explained to the patient and the family members prior to surgery. (**h**) In this patient, the degenerative stromal lesion reached the margin of the pupil; thus, pterygium surgery did not successfully restore the cosmetic appearance or improve the vision

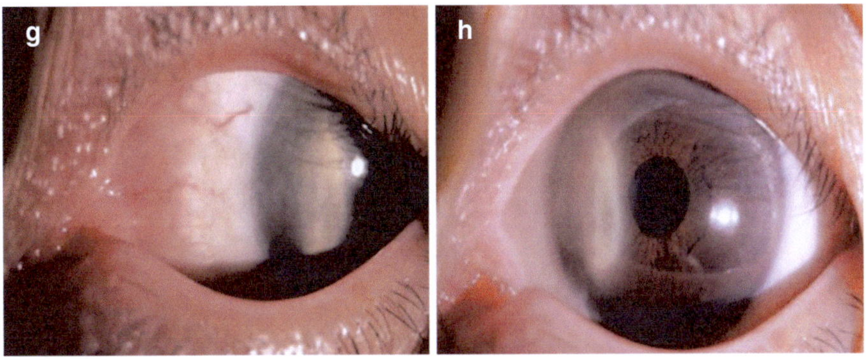

Fig. 3.10 (continued)

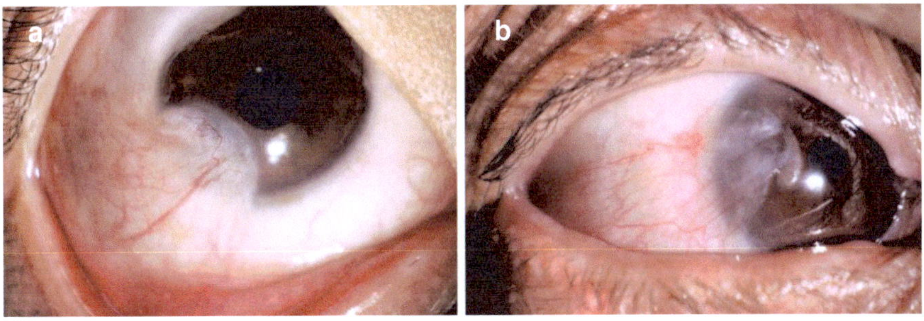

Fig. 3.11 (**a**, **b**) Temporal pterygium

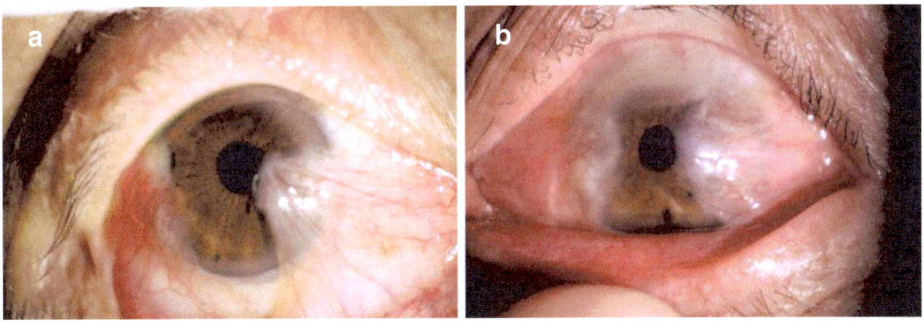

Fig. 3.12 (**a**, **b**) Double pterygium: pterygium grows simultaneously on both the nasal and temporal sides of the same eye

3. **Invasive pterygium** The growth of invasive pterygium is similar to horizontal pterygium, this type of pterygium is classified as primary pterygium. Because during the development the head of pterygium breaks either through Bowman's layer or invades the superficial stroma tissue of the cornea, due to these tissue cannot be fully surgically separated and removed. Consequently, not only pterygium infiltration causes an uneven corneal surface, but also the pterygium residue embedded into the stroma tissue is difficult to remove, even with a small

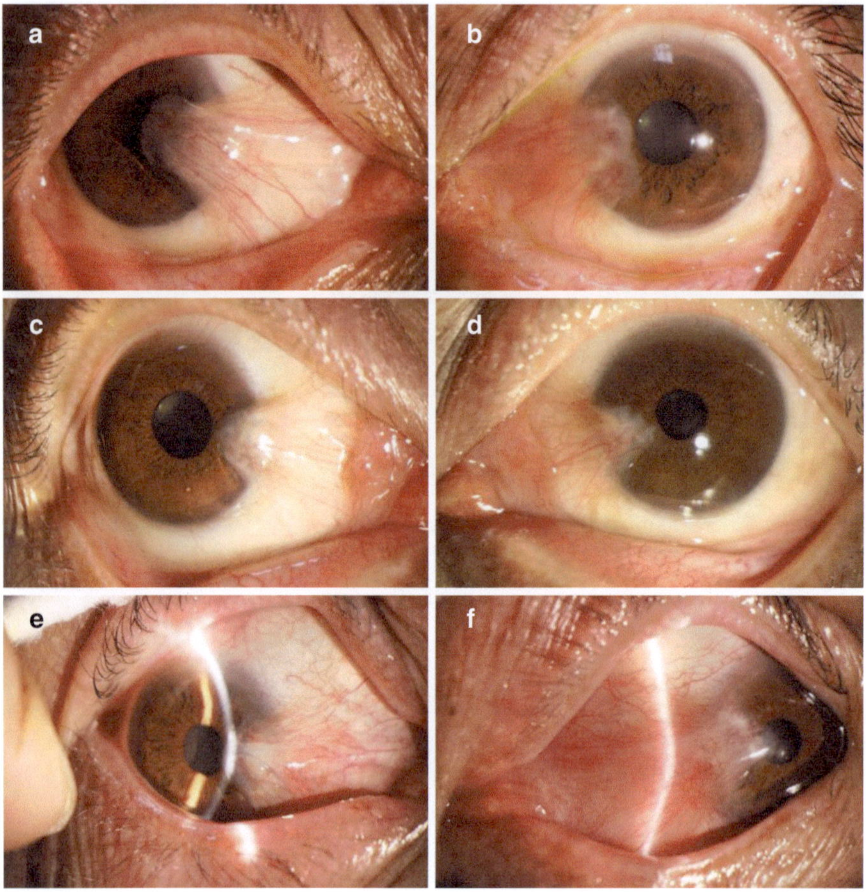

Fig. 3.13 Bilateral pterygium. (**a**, **b**) Showed a patient, who had pterygium in both eyes; (**c**, **d**) showed a patient, had pterygium in both eyes; (**e**, **f**) showed a patient, who had pterygium in both eyes

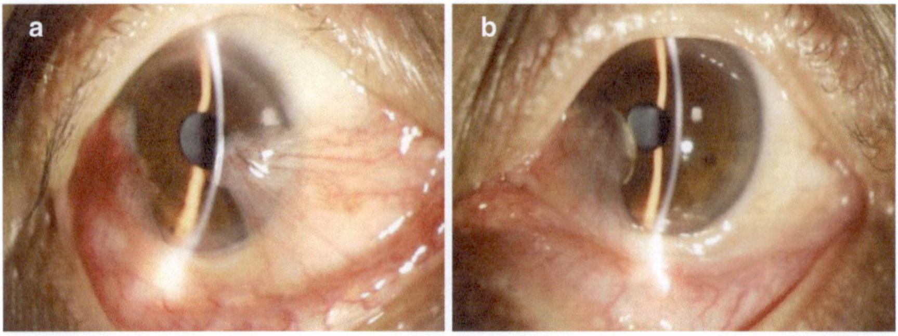

Fig. 3.14 (**a**, **b**) Bilateral double pterygium. In the eyes of a patient with double pterygium in right eye and single pterygium in left eye

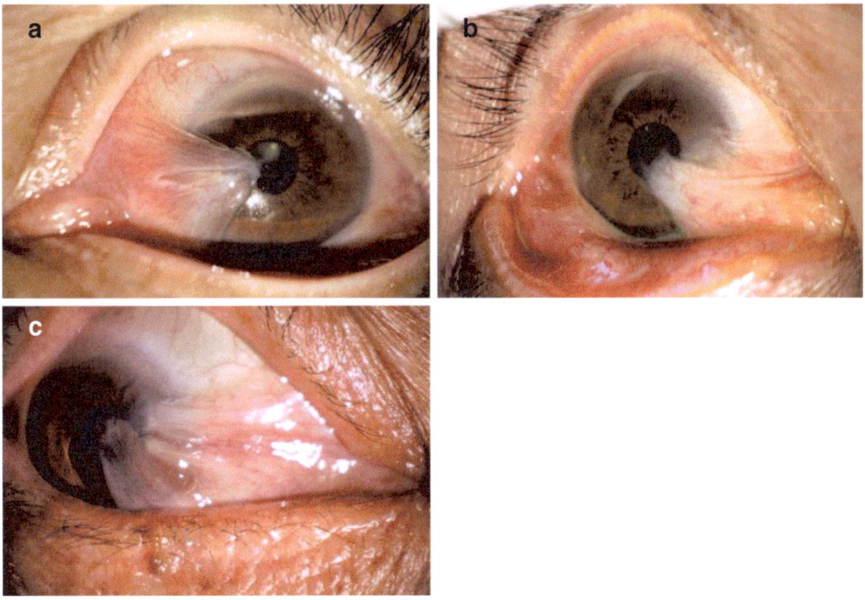

Fig. 3.15 Double-headed and multiheaded pterygium. (**a**) Double-headed pterygium: pterygium has two heads, making the corneal wound surface difficult to manage during surgery. (**b**) Multiheaded pterygium: for pterygium with three heads, it is likely that a very small amount of pterygium tissue may remain on the corneal wound after surgery. This situation should be explained to the patient prior to surgery, and this type of pterygium surgery should not be performed by an inexperienced surgeon. (**c**) Multiheaded pterygium: for pterygium with four heads, it is likely that a very small amount of pterygium tissue will remain on the corneal wound after surgery. This situation should be explained to the patient prior to surgery, and this type of pterygium surgery should not be performed by an unexperienced surgeon

circular blade or grinding tool. This type of surgery is a challenge, especially to beginner surgeons.

When removing residual part of the pterygium, inexperienced surgeons often damage the corneal stroma, resulting in the delayed healing of the corneal epithelium or the perforation of the stroma. This situation should pay special attention during surgery. It is unnecessary to treat the small amount of residual pterygium tissue at the corneal limbus due to that does not affect the visual axis of the pupil (Fig. 3.18).

Infiltrative pterygium has the following characteristics. First, the pterygium head is wide and invades the corneal stroma. Second, infiltrative pterygium occurs mostly among young people and is often actively growing. Surgery for infiltrative pterygium should not be performed by a beginner surgeon.

3.1.3.2 Characteristics of Pterygium at Different Stages

Primary pterygium can be categorized into three stages: active stage, stationary stage, and regressive stage [1].

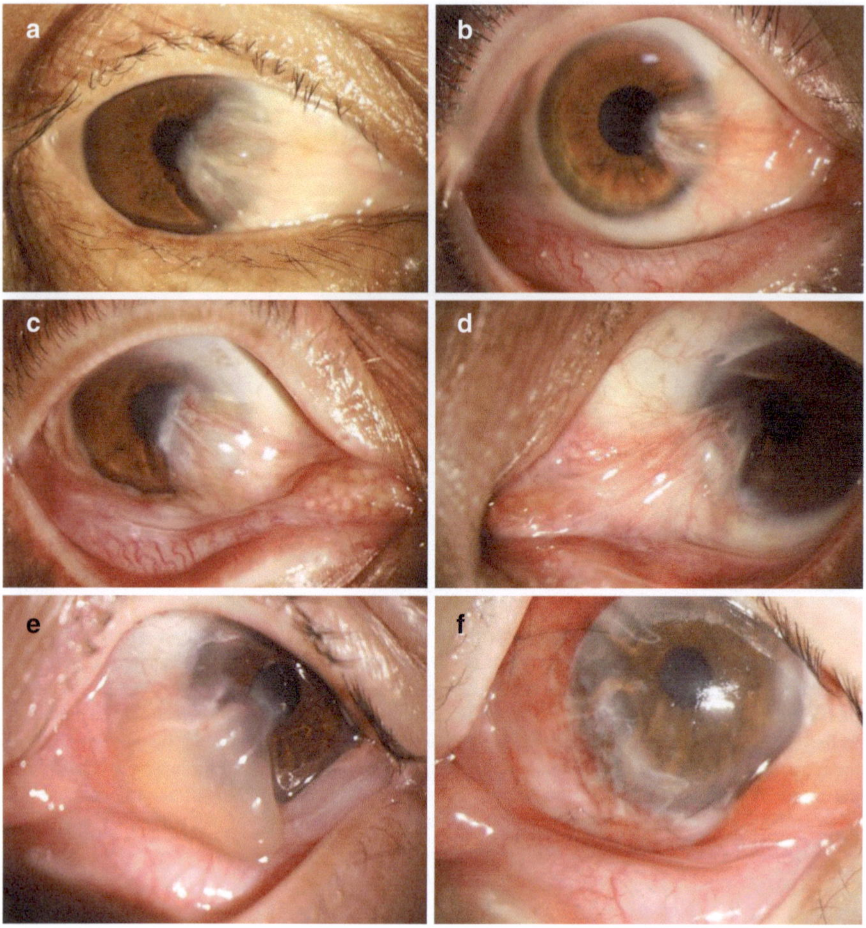

Fig. 3.16 Pterygium with conjunctival cysts. (**a**) For primary pterygium with multiple conjunctival cysts on the head, the cysts should be surgically removed together with the pterygium and pathologically examined; cysts are generally benign. (**b**) Pterygium with a single small conjunctival cyst on the neck. (**c**) Pterygium with a single large conjunctival cyst on the neck. (**d**) For primary pterygium with a conjunctival cyst on its neck, the cyst should be surgically removed together with the pterygium and pathologically examined. (**e**) Giant conjunctival cysts that involve the pterygium head, neck, and body should be surgically removed together with the pterygium and pathologically examined. (**f**) A photo of a pterygium patient with a giant cyst (**e**) on the second day after surgery

1. **Active stage** Pterygium at this stage is actively growing with enlarged blood vessels and is often hypertrophic with severe congestion. Surgery can be performed only after inflammation has been effectively controlled by anti-inflammatory treatment or has completely subsided (Fig. 3.19).
2. **Quiescent pterygium** The head part of the pterygium is pale, the blood vessels are fine and small, and the growth is stopped, which is the best period for surgery (Fig. 3.20).
3. **Regressive stage** Regressive pterygium has a thin body and a pale head. The surgical approach should be selected on the basis of the patient's needs (Fig. 3.21).

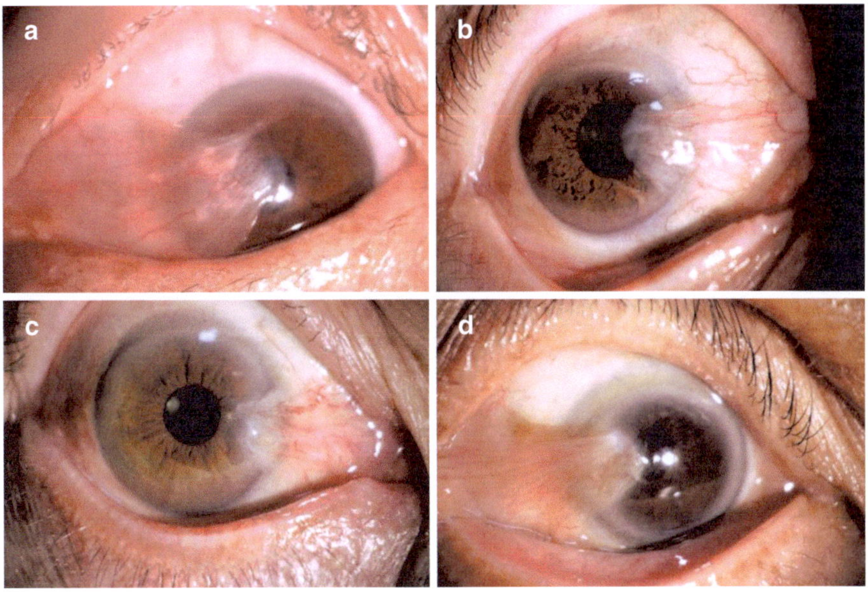

Fig. 3.17 Horizontal grow type of pterygium. (**a–d**) Pterygium is at the static phase, with the head attached to the corneal epithelium, and the excision is adequate for beginners to perform

3.1.4 Laboratory Examination

No evidence is available showing that primary pterygium causes changes in laboratory blood tests. However, studies have been reported about the changes in the conjunctival sac of patients with primary pterygium, including an increase in eosinophils, changes in impression cytology, an increase in tear osmolality, and inflammatory cell activation. These are dry eye-related changes might be induced by pterygium-caused dry eye but not pterygium itself.

3.1.5 Diagnosis and Differential Diagnosis

3.1.5.1 Diagnosis

The main diagnostic criterion for primary pterygium include the following:

1. History: The patient could present with or without a family history of pterygium, with or without history of ocular or systemic immune disease, ocular trauma (including chemical injury), or ocular infectious disease. The patient may have a long history of pinguecula.

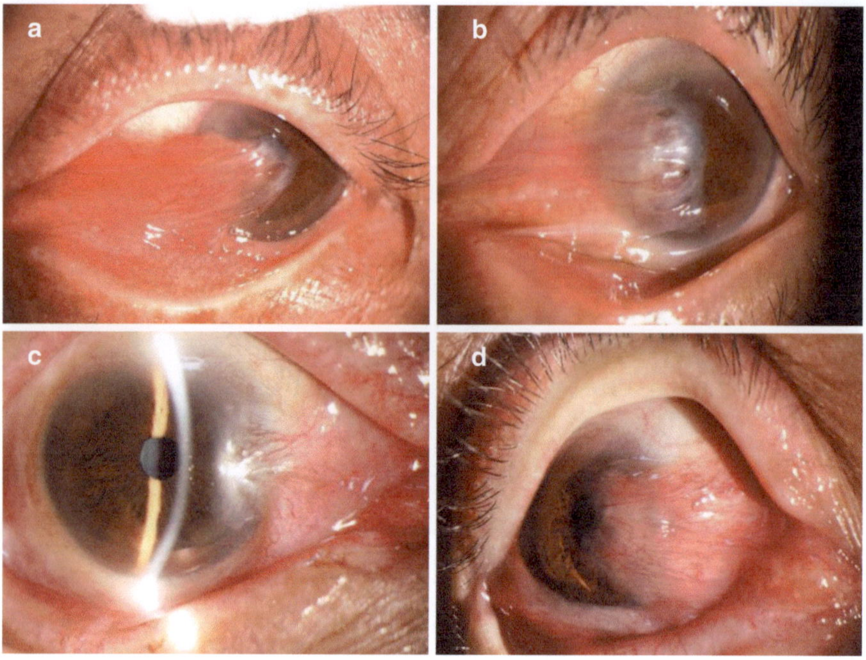

Fig. 3.18 Infiltrative pterygium. (**a**) The pterygium head is wide and invades the corneal stroma. Pterygium is actively growing with serious congestion. Surgery can be performed only after inflammation is controlled. It is likely that there will be some pterygium tissue residue and the corneal wound surface is uneven after surgery. (**b**) The pterygium head is wide and invades the corneal stroma. The patient received 3 days of anti-inflammatory treatment. It is difficult to completely remove the pterygium, and it is likely that the corneal surface affected will be uneven after surgery. Therefore, the surgery should not be performed by a beginner surgeon. (**c**) The pterygium head is wide and invades the corneal stroma. (**d**) The pterygium head is wide and invades into the corneal stroma

2. Signs: An unexplained, painless proliferative fibrovascular membrane arising from the interpalpebral fissure conjunctiva gradually extends to the cornea. The signs of primary pterygium are as follows:
    (a) Growth at 3 or 9 o'clock of the interpalpebral conjunctival zone;
    (b) It could be divided into three clear parts, i.e., head, neck, and body;
    (c) Adherence of the neck to the scleral tissue at the corneal limbus, where a surgical probe cannot pass through.

3.1.5.2 Differential Diagnosis

Primary pterygium should be distinguished from the following diseases.

1. Pinguecula:

    Pinguecula is a light yellowish, raised growth on the interpalpebral bulbar conjunctiva. It is limited to the interpalpebral conjunctiva, mostly the nasal side,

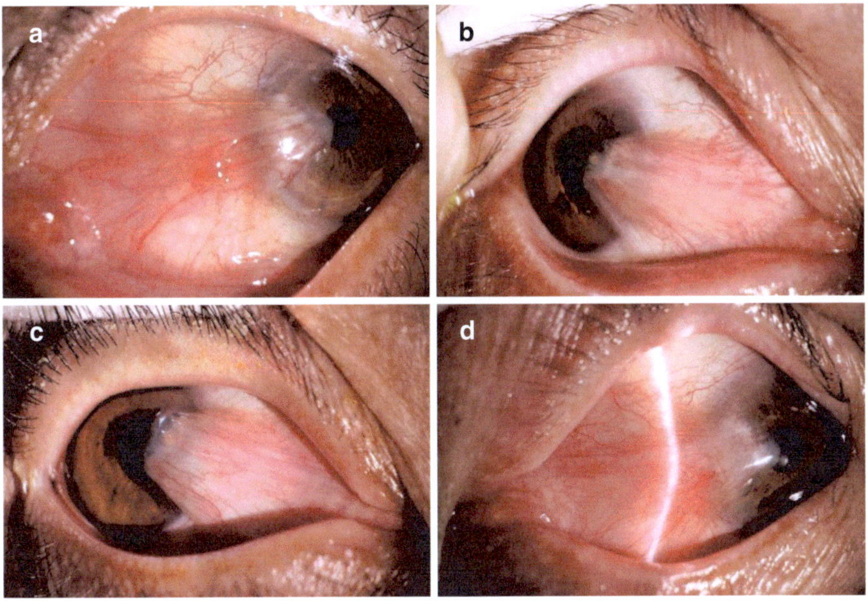

Fig. 3.19 Active stage of pterygium. (**a–d**) The growth of pterygium is active, the blood vessels are thick, tissue hypertrophy. Topical anti-inflammatory therapy with glucocorticoids should be used before surgery, and surgery should be performed after congestion is reduced or inflammation subsides, which can reduce postoperative complications and recurrence

without affecting the cornea. Pinguecula occurs more often in people living in lake areas, by the sea, or in high-altitude areas where UV irradiation is strong. There is evidence indicating that a considerable proportion of primary pterygium develops from long term pinguecula that invades the cornea.

In 1869, Zehender first proposed that pinguecula was a precursor to pterygium. This theory was supported by Fuchs, Parsons, and Alt [1], but without solid data evidence to confirm. The symptoms of pinguecula are the same as those of primary pterygium, including eye dryness, foreign body sensation, eye itchiness, and eye swelling; cosmetic disturbance may occur if the pinguecula is large (Figs. 3.22 and 3.23).

2. Conjunctival papilloma:

   Conjunctival papillomas located at the corneal limbus are reddish, round, granular, and raised lesions. Large conjunctival papillomas may cover the corneal surface near the corneal limbus but do not invade the cornea. Conjunctival papillomas do not have a structure consisting of a head, neck, and body, which can be differentiated from **primary pterygium** (Fig. 3.24**).**

3. **Pseudo Pterygium:**

   It is growing from surface of the eyeball, commonly from chemical burn, hot burn, mechanical burn injury of the eyeball, scarring conjunctivitis and immunogenic infection disease of surface of the eyeball (see the third section). Characteristic of pseudo pterygium are: (1)unlike primary pterygium only growing at 3 o'clock and/or 9 o'clock bulbal conjunctival in the lid fis-

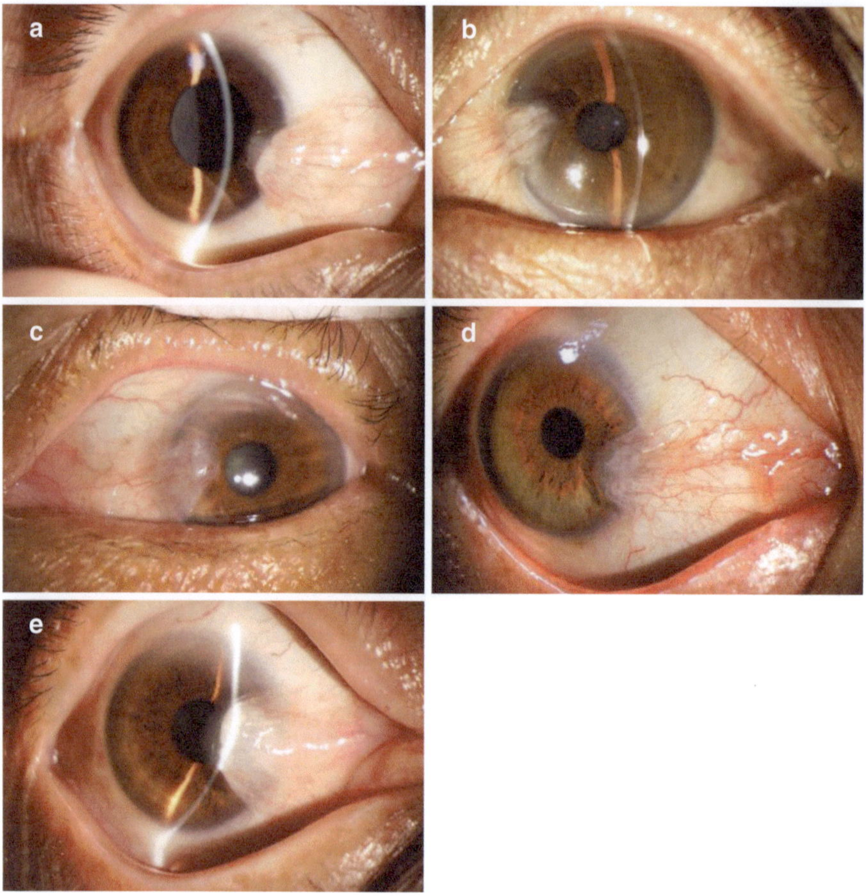

Fig. 3.20 Quiescent pterygium. (**a**–**e**) The head part of the pterygium is pale, the blood vessels are fine and small, and the growth is stopped, which is the best period for surgery

sure area. (2) Without could be identified the portion of head, neck, and body. (3) Pseudo pterygium from limbus of the cornea but not adhesion to sclera, probing can be passed underneath (Table 3.1).

Corneal SCC is a primary malignancy of the ocular surface in the interpalpebral area and occurs mostly among middle-aged and elderly individuals. The tumour has a wide base on the corneal limbus, similar to pterygium, but its tip grows towards the conjunctiva. The tumour often breaks through the basement membrane, and its surface is cauliflower-shaped and bleeds easily when touched. A corneal SCC does not have a structure consisting of a head, neck, and body, which is unique to primary pterygium, and can be distinguished from primary pterygium via pathological examination of the lesion (Fig. 3.25).

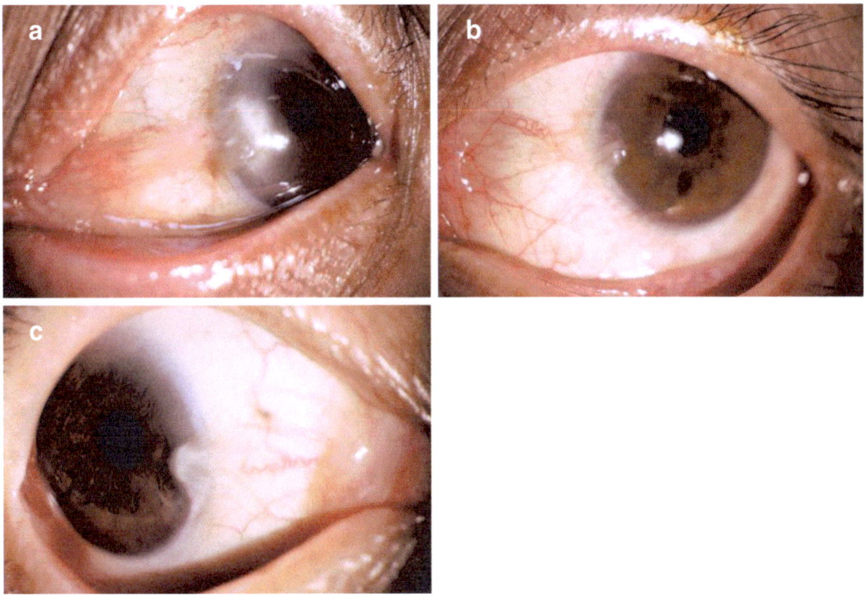

Fig. 3.21 Degenerative pterygium. (**a–c**) The body part of the pterygium is thin and the head part of the pterygium is pale, and ordinary pterygium surgery is allowed

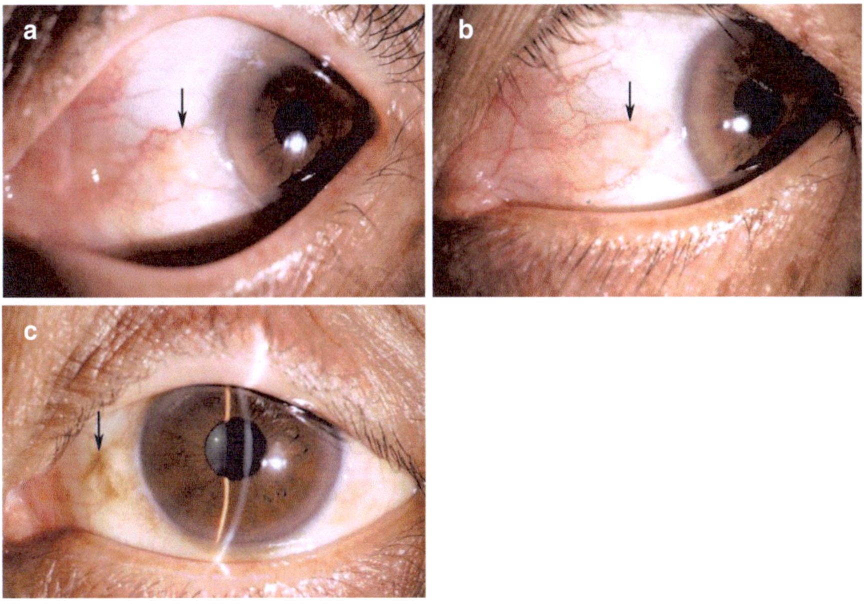

Fig. 3.22 Pinguecula. (**a–c**) Pinguecula is a pale yellowish, raised growth on the interpalpebral bulbar conjunctiva (black arrow) and does not invade the cornea

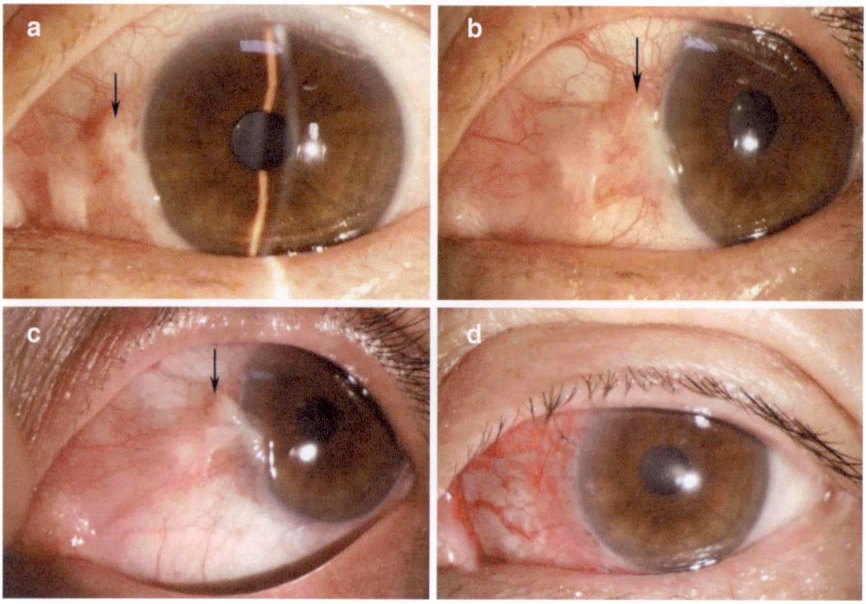

Fig. 3.23 A patient whose pterygium developed from pinguecula and was surgically treated. (**a**, **b**) A photo taken on October 9, 2017, showing that the pinguecula did not invade the cornea (black arrow). (**c**) A photo taken during a follow-up visit on December 2, 2019, showing that the pinguecula grew into the corneal limbus and formed a primary pterygium (black arrow). The patient requested surgery to improve cosmetic appearance. (**d**) A photo taken the day after surgery

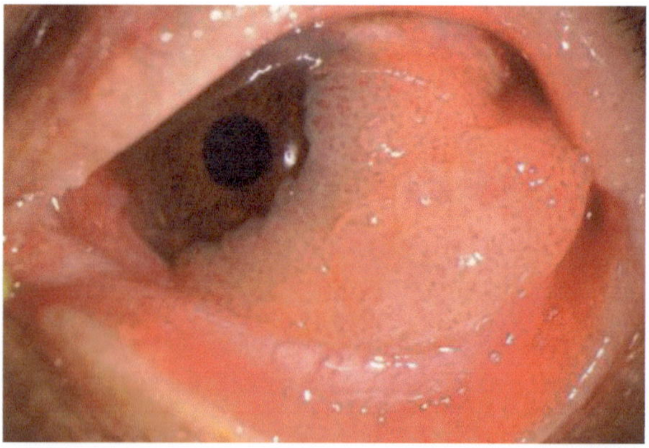

Fig. 3.24 Conjunctival papilloma covers corneal lesions the eminence is reddish, granular and round mass

4. Recurrent pterygium is the results from post operation or several operations pterygium regrow through the limbus into the cornea. According to the location of regrowth tissue invading into the corneal and whether it is accompanied with symblepharon, recurrent pterygium can be classified (see Sect. 3.3 for details):

Table 3.1 Key points to differentiate true pterygium from pseudo pterygium

–	True pterygium	Pseudopterygium
Cause	Physical stimulation or chronic inflammation	Ulcers, burns, and chemical injuries of the corneal limbus
Location	Occurs on the nasal and temporal conjunctiva at the interpalpebral fissure and invades the cornea to varying extents	Occurs any location in the cornea
Growth pattern	Expands towards the central cornea; congested and accompanied with chronic inflammation	Does not progress; no congestion and inflammation
Examination with a probe	Probe cannot pass through the area underneath the neck of pterygium	Probe can pass through underneath the neck of pterygium

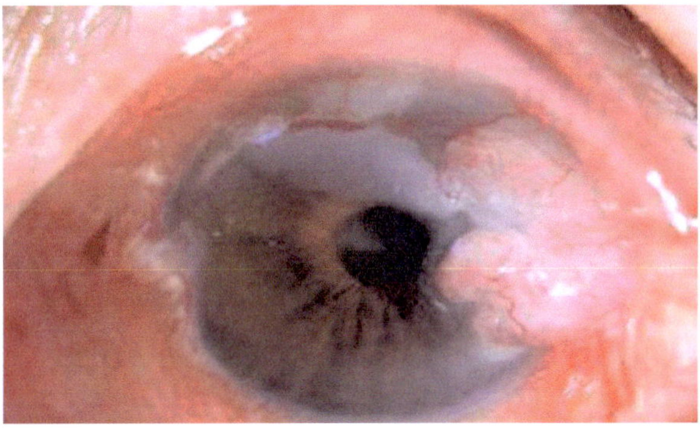

Fig. 3.25 Corneal squamous cell carcinoma

(a) Mild recurrent pterygium: pterygium infiltrates into the corneal limbus less than 1 mm.
(b) Moderate recurrent pterygium: pterygium infiltrates into the corneal limbus by 1–3 mm without symblepharon.
(c) Severe recurrent: Recurrent pterygium infiltrates into the corneal limbus more than 3 mm, accompanied by symblepharon [1].

3.2 Section 2: Clinical Features of Recurrent Pterygium

Recurrent pterygium refers to pterygium regrowth after resection of the primary pterygium and has the following clinical characteristics:

1. It is fibrovascular growth tissue with poor elasticity;
2. Fibrovascular tissue often simultaneously grow into the corneal stroma, superficial sclera, and Tenon's capsule;

3. Scar tissue formation may involve the medial rectus muscle sheath, upper and lower eyelids, and lacrimal caruncle; potentially induce severe symblepharon limiting the eye movement and causes severe diplopia;
4. After multiple recurrences, invasion towards the cornea reaching the pupil area, with the potential to cover the pupil, can lead to blindness in the affected eye and seriously affect visual function (Fig. 3.26, 3.27, 3.28, 3.29, 3.30, and 3.31).

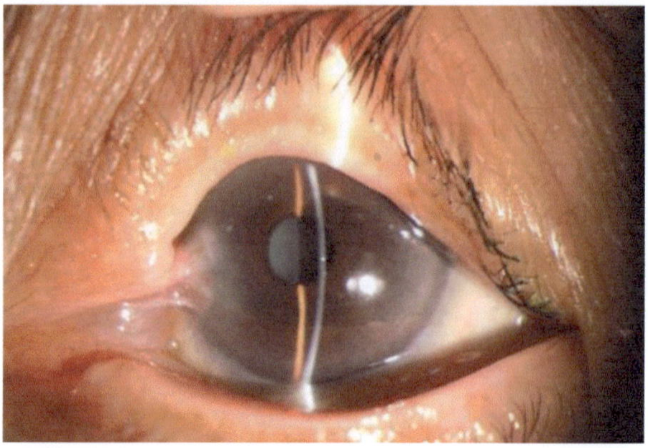

Fig. 3.26 Recurrent pterygium. After three times of pterygium operations without under the surgical microscope were performed at several local hospitals. At meantime the secondary recurrence, the nasal upper eyelid conjunctiva on the with recurrent pterygium adheres to the cornea, showing oculomotor dyskinesia and severe diplopia

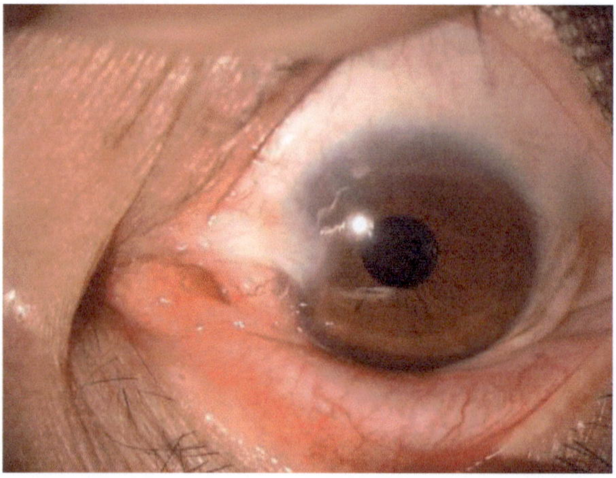

Fig. 3.27 Recurrent pterygium. A 36-year-old patient with recurrent pterygium after 4 non-microscopic surgeries done in a local township hospital, showing nasal symblepharon, the eyeball fixed on nasal side, dyskinesia, severe diplopia, and no ability to do normal work

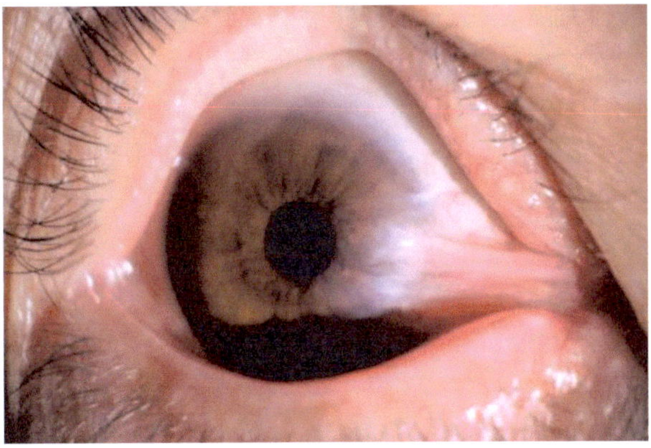

Fig. 3.28 This patient with three non-microscopic surgeries for pterygium operation, but recurrent pterygium was still occurred. Therefore post-operative period pterygium recurred causes symblepharon oculomotor dyskinesia and diplopia

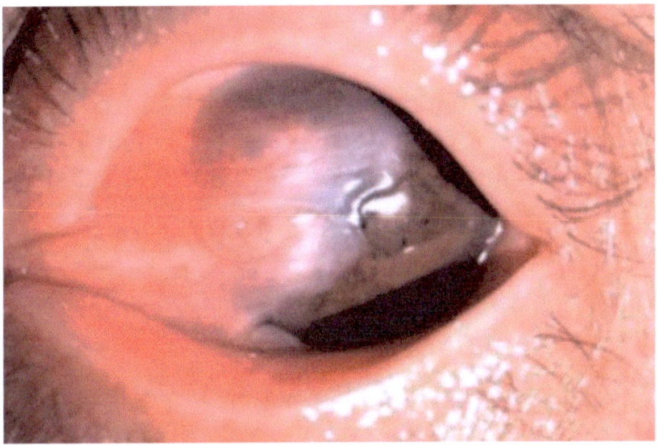

Fig. 3.29 Recurrent pterygium covers the pupil and caused blindness

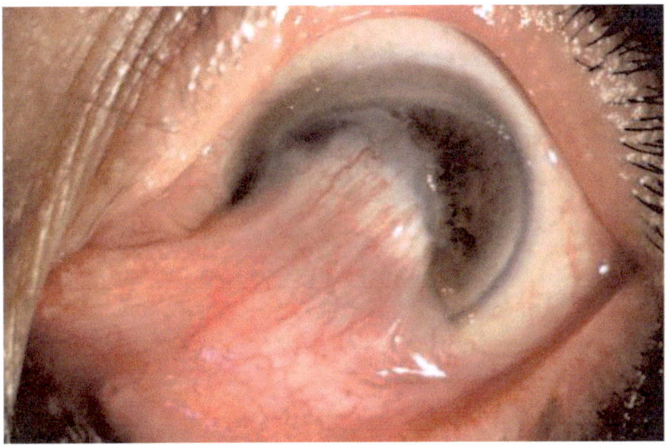

Fig. 3.30 A patient had two surgeries for recurrent pterygium reoccurred, which covers the pupil and visual acuity reduced to hand movement

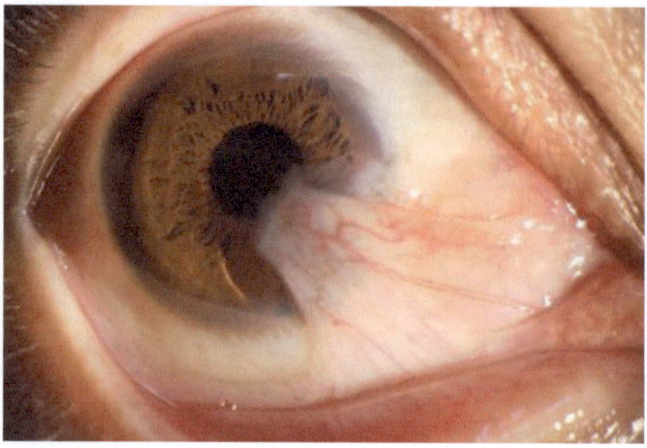

Fig. 3.31 A patient with recurrent pterygium after microsurgery, symblepharon is not severe, but more than 3 mm lacrimal caruncle is displaced

3.3 Section 3: Clinical Features of Pseudopterygium

Pseudopterygium refers to a conjunctival fold resulting from the adhesion of an acutely injured cornea at the corneal limbus to the nearby bulbar conjunctiva after acute injury [2] (Figs. 3.32, 3.33, 3.34, 3.35, 3.36, 3.37, 3.38, and 3.39).

3.3.1 Common Causes of Pseudopterygium

1. Mechanical trauma to the eye that is not treated properly in a timely manner.
2. Marginal corneal ulceration, especially Mooren's ulcer.
3. Complications from an ocular surface chemical injury.
4. Severe dry eye due to ocular surface autoimmune disorders.
5. Infectious ocular surface disease.

3.3.2 Clinical Features of Pseudopterygium

1. **The location of Pseudopterygium** is not limited to the interpalpebral fissure; instead, it may occur at any corneal meridian.
2. From underneath a pseudopterygium, a surgical probe can be passed through along to the opposite corneal limbus.
3. Pseudopterygium often occurs unilaterally.
4. Pseudopterygium can regress after treatment of the primary disease is controlled.

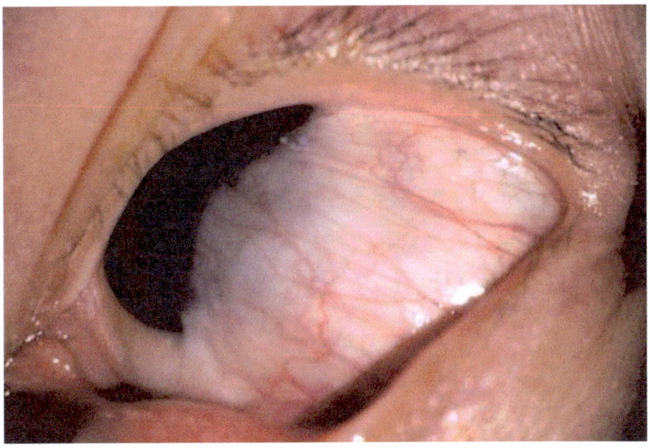

Fig. 3.32 Chemical injury complicated by pseudopterygium injury. At 0.5–1 year after injury, corneal limbus stem cell transplantation is first performed, and subsequent treatment is determined according to postoperative ocular surface recovery

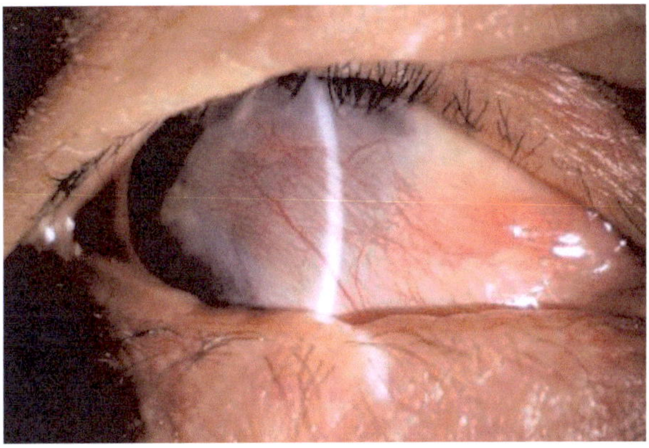

Fig. 3.33 Chemical injury complicated with pseudopterygium. 0.5–1 year after injury, corneal limbus stem cell transplantation is first choice to performed, and the subsequent treatment is determine according to postoperative ocular surface recovery

5. Pseudopterygium caused by chemical injury is often associated with damage to the limbus Stem cells (LSCs); therefore, treatment requires ocular surface reconstruction or LSC transplantation, which should be implemented by multiple surgeries.
6. For pseudopterygium caused by mechanical trauma, a proper surgical approach should be selected based on the location and degree of damage.
7. Pseudopterygium is not primary pterygium; hence, conventional pterygium surgical approaches might not be suitable for pseudopterygium.

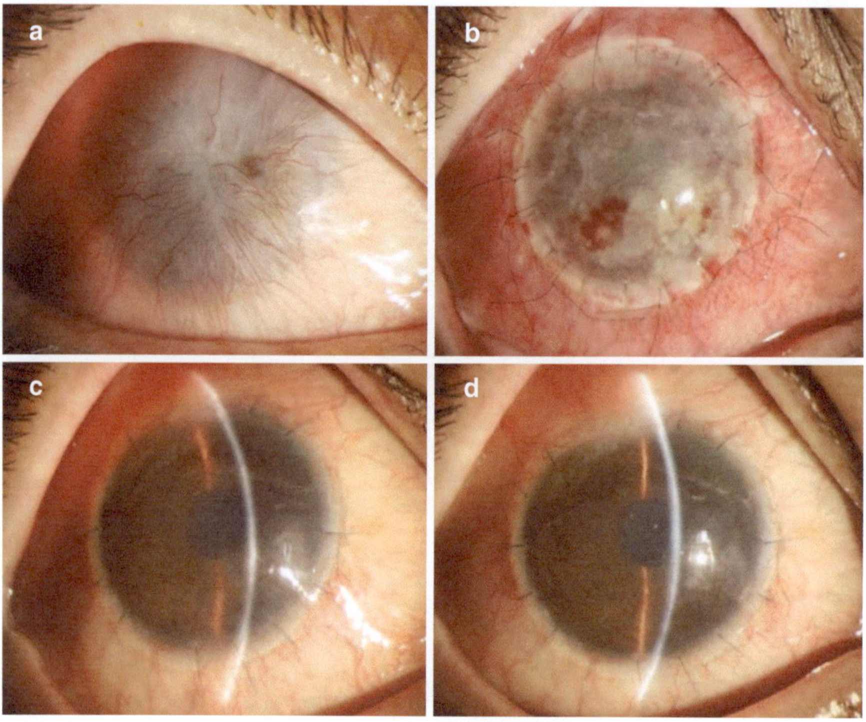

Fig. 3.34 Pre- and postoperative photo of a case of pseudopterygium. (**a**) Two years after an alkali burn, pseudopterygium covered the corneal surface, with symblepharon at the upper part of the eyeball and a white plaque in the center. (**b**) The patient received anterior lamellar keratoplasty (ALK) with allogeneic limbal stem cell transplant and had an uncorrected visual acuity of 0.06 on the second day after surgery. (**c**) The patient had a visual acuity of 0.25 on the 51st day after surgery. Neovascularization of the graft bed partially subsided, and epithelial repaired. (**d**) On the 83rd day after surgery, the visual acuity was 0.5, and neovascularization of the graft bed had mostly subsided. Superior symblepharon was disappeared and eyeball movements returned to normal

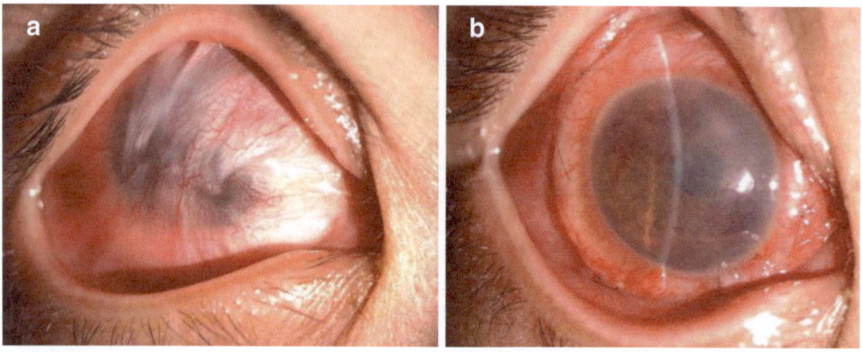

Fig. 3.35 Pre- and postoperative photo of a case of pseudopterygium. (**a**) Lime burn of the eye complicated by pseudopterygium before surgery. (**b**) Seven days after ocular surface reconstruction, the patient had an uncorrected visual acuity of 0.1

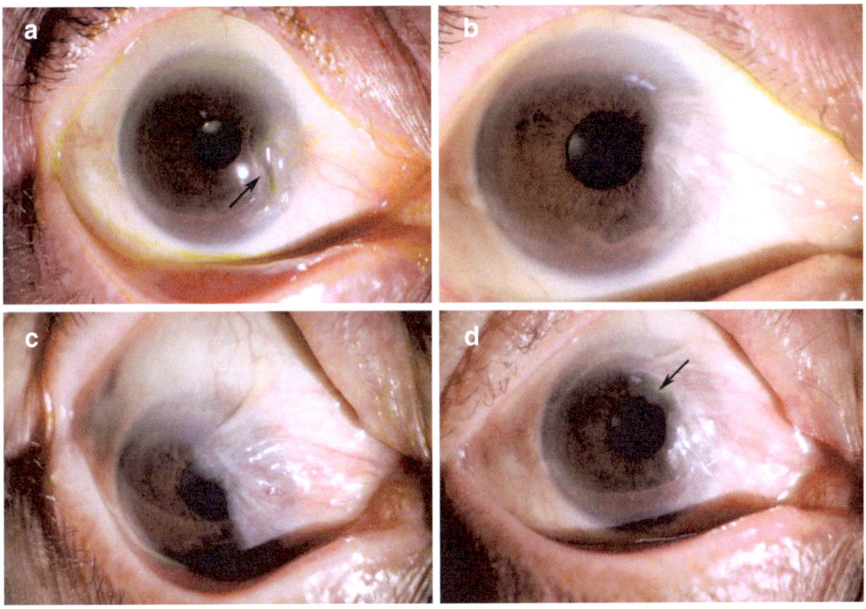

Fig. 3.36 Progression of a pseudopterygium associated with Mooren's corneal ulcer. (**a**) Pseudopterygium covered the lesioned area surrounding the furrow of Mooren's ulcer (black arrow) (photo taken in 2015). For this type of pseudopterygium, conventional pterygium surgery is not suitable, and instead, anti-immunotherapy is indicated. (**b**) Pseudopterygium covered the furrow of Mooren's ulcer, easily leading to a misdiagnosis as primary pterygium (photo taken in 2016). A detailed medical history of the patient is essential. (**c**) Three years later, pseudopterygium tissue adhesion was present, and nonsurgical treatment was the only option (photo taken in September 2019). (**d**) Mooren's ulcer re-occurred on the limbus of the cornea at 2 o'clock on the pseudopterygium (black arrow), and medication remained the only treatment option

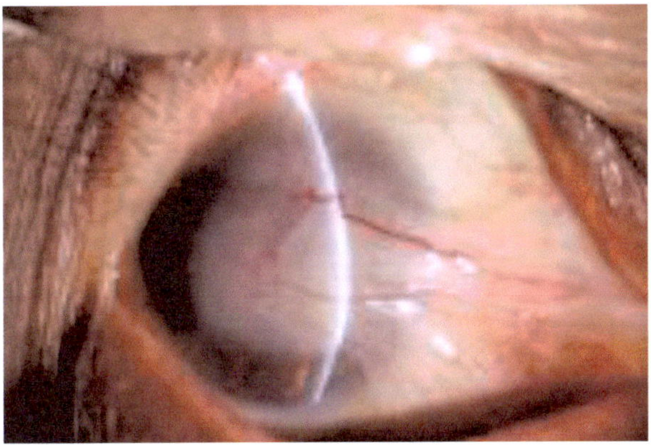

Fig. 3.37 Herpes simplex keratitis (HSK)with pseudopterygium. The central cornea of the patient had disciform stromal opacity, and the conjunctiva was "pulled" to the centre of the lesion. Endothelial cell morphology and counting should be used to determine whether such patients should be treated with deep lamellar keratoplasty or penetrating keratoplasty (PKP)

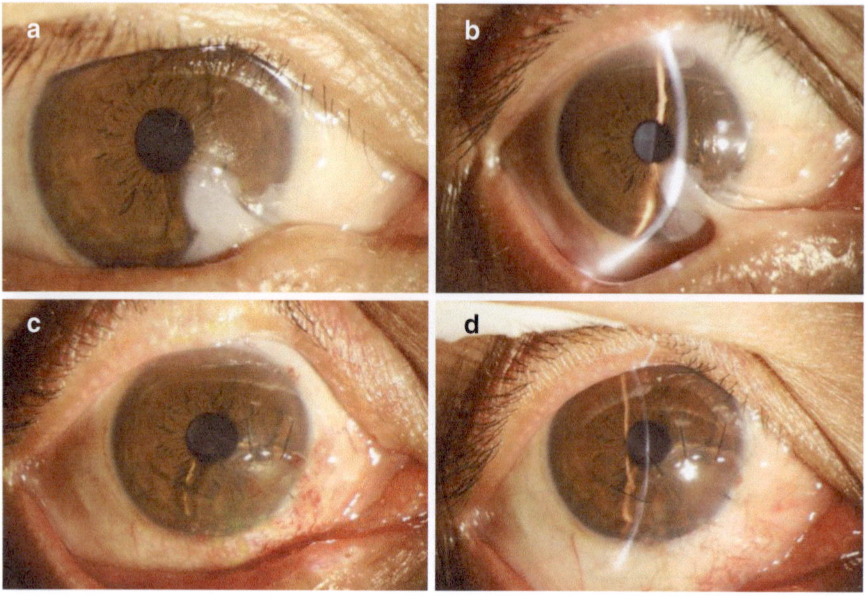

Fig. 3.38 A case of mechanical ocular trauma (wounded by a bamboo pierce) complicated with pseudopterygium in pre and after operation. (**a**) Pseudopterygium was located at the 5 o'clock position. (**b**) Inferior symblepharon could be clearly seen when pulling the lower eyelid down, and eye movements were restricted. (**c**) Two weeks after partial lamellar keratoplasty, the patient had deteriorated visual acuity (worsened by two rows); surgery was performed after the patient was fully aware of and understood the situation. (**d**) The symblepharon was released, and eye movements returned to normal after surgery

Fig. 3.39 Steven-Johnson syndrome complicated with pseudopterygium. The patient was 17 years old. Normal limbal palisades of Vogt were absent. The patient was treated mainly with nonsurgical approaches

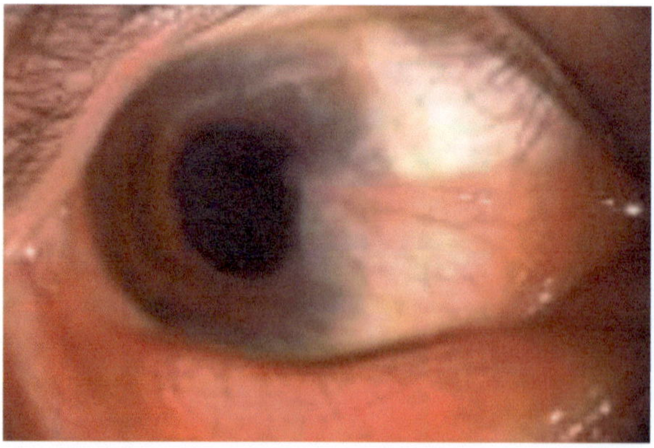

3.4 Section 4: Prevention and Treatment of Pterygium

3.4.1 Prevention

Because the aetiology and pathogenesis of pterygium is unknown, it is difficult to develop effective measures for prevention. In addition to genetic factors, epidemiological surveys of pterygium have revealed a high incidence rate among residents living in areas that have a high UV light and/or sunlight exposure, are at high altitude, or have dusty, windy/sandy, and dry environments. Therefore, theoretically, reducing or limiting sunlight exposure and avoiding working in a dusty, windy/sandy, and dry environment could prevent the occurrence of pterygium.

Gamerron et al. had found that the incidence of pterygium in Australia decreased from an average of 15% to 3% among people who consistently wore glasses before the age of 5. Mackenzie et al. stated that healthy people who did not wear glasses regularly had a threefold higher risk of developing pterygium than those who often wore glasses. When exposed to sunlight, the occurrence of pterygium was five times higher among the general population than among those who wore dark sunglasses. The correlation between sunlight and the occurrence of pterygium was also demonstrated in a study that compared people who wore and do not wear hats in sunlight. Therefore, Mackenzie et al. recommended avoiding exposure to UV light, especially before the age of 5 [1]. Some researchers believe that the development of pterygium is associated with allergic conjunctivitis, dry eyes, and immune-mediated conjunctival inflammation and that proper treatment and management of these diseases can prevent the occurrence of pterygium [2].

3.4.2 Treatment

3.4.2.1 Nonsurgical Treatment

Primary pterygium itself cannot be effectively treated by medication, but drugs can be used to alleviate pterygium-caused eye discomfort, such as dry eye, foreign body sensation, and eye redness. In addition, drugs that are used to treat allergies and immune disorders might delay the progression of pterygium because of a possible association of primary pterygium with allergies and immunity. However, the efficacy of these treatments has not been proven by statistical data.

1. **Anti-inflammatory drugs** Anti-inflammatory drugs can be applied to control the active inflammatory response in the active stage of pterygium. In addition, dry eye, which is caused by the combination of tear kinetic abnormalities resulting from pterygium bulging from the conjunctival surface and lipid abnormalities resulting from wind/sand disturbances and UV radiation, can result in inflammation. Hence, anti-inflammatory drugs should be considered as a treatment option for pterygium. Common glucocorticoid steroids used locally for

short-term treatment at low doses to alleviate symptoms and control inflammation are 0.5% loteprednol etabonate and 0.1% fluorometholone.

2. **Antimetabolites** Pterygium is identified as a proliferative disease. Antimetabolites, including mitomycin C (MMC), fluorouracil (5-Fu), and pingyangmycin, have been proposed by some researchers to prevent the proliferation of fibrovascular tissue and elastic fibres growth. Direct injection of the drug into the pterygium body to reduce the size of the pterygium. However, antimetabolites are highly toxic and may have unpredictable complications when used locally; therefore, they must be used with caution [2].
3. **Artificial tears** Dry eye caused by pterygium is often the mixed type and mostly moderate. Artificial tears combined with the short-term use of anti-inflammatory drugs can temporarily relieve dry eye symptoms.
4. **Cryotherapy and laser treatment** Cryotherapy using a −40 °C cryo probe to directly contact the pterygium head and neck may shrink the pterygium. This method is simple and has very few side effects, but it does not prevent pterygium recurrence. In addition, small pterygium can be excised with YAG lasers, CO_2 lasers, excimer lasers, etc., which use the thermal effect of laser irradiation to block the blood supply and thus shrink the pterygium [2].
5. **Aprotinin** Aprotinin can significantly inhibit the hydrogen peroxide-induced secretion of TNF-α by pterygium fibroblasts. Research has shown that TNF-α plays an important role in the formation and recurrence of pterygium. Hence, aprotinin might be a novel promising drug for pterygium prevention and treatment [2].

3.4.2.2 Surgical Treatment (See Part III Surgery)

References

1. Foster CS, Azar DT, Dohlman CH. Smolin and Thoft's the cornea: scientific foundations and clinical practice (Chinese version translated by Li Y). Tianjin: Tianjin Science & Technology Translation & Publishing Corp.; 2007. p. 987–1001.
2. Xie LX. Atlas of corneal disease. Beijing: People's Medical Publishing House; 2011. p. 368–73.

Part III
Surgical Treatment

Chapter 4
Surgical indications and Evaluation

Hansheng Liu, Congxiang Wang, and Kuanshu Li

4.1 Section 1: Surgical Purposes and Main Factors Affecting Surgical Decision-Making

4.1.1 Surgical Purposes

4.1.1.1 Visual Improvement

When pterygium causes obvious corneal astigmatism or covers the pupil, blurred vision, decreased vision, or even blindness can occur, thus seriously affecting the reading ability and quality of life of patients, which may require surgical treatment (Figs. 4.1 and 4.2).

4.1.1.2 Cosmetic Improvement

Pterygium, which is located in the interpalpebral area and invades the corneal limbus, may obviously affect appearance, and active pterygium may also cause redness of the eye. The cosmetic disturbance caused by pterygium might limit patients' social activities. With improvements in living standards, elderly people in the countryside have begun to have higher requirements regarding the cosmetic appearance of the eyes. Hence, the cosmetic outcome of pterygium surgery has attracted

H. Liu (✉)
Medical Management Center, Aier Eye Hospital Group, Changsha, China

C. Wang · K. Li (✉)
Changsha Aier Eye Hospital, Changsha, China

C. Wang, S. Li (eds.), *Pterygium Surgery*,
https://doi.org/10.1007/978-981-99-6843-5_4

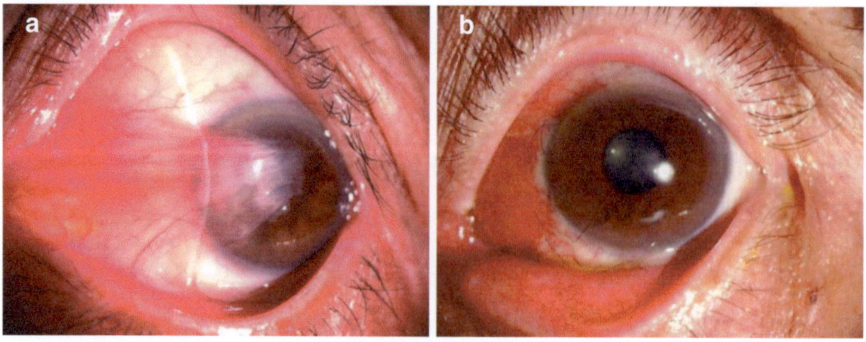

Fig. 4.1 Giant pterygium before and after surgery. (**a**) A giant pterygium covered the pupil area and caused blindness. The patient's visual acuity was "hand movement (HM) in front of the eye." (**b**) The patient's visual acuity improved to 0.6 on the second postoperative day

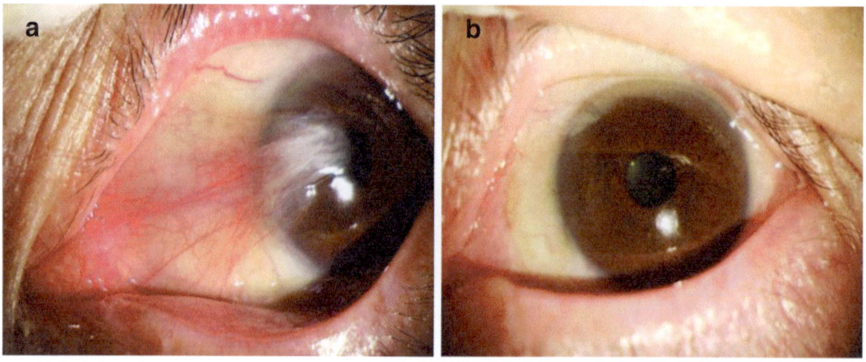

Fig. 4.2 Pterygium before and after surgery. (**a**) Pterygium partially covered the pupil area. The patient's uncorrected visual acuity was 0.2. (**b**) The patient's uncorrected visual acuity improved to 1.0 at 1 year and 5 months postoperatively

attention from professionals in this field and has been considered a key criterion for evaluating surgical success (Figs. 4.3, 4.4, and 4.5).

4.1.1.3 Improvement of Eye Discomfort Symptoms

The main causes of pterygium-related eye discomfort include mixed-type dry eye, symblepharon that limits eye movements, immune inflammatory responses, and corneal astigmatism that causes blurred vision (Figs. 4.6, 4.7, and 4.8).

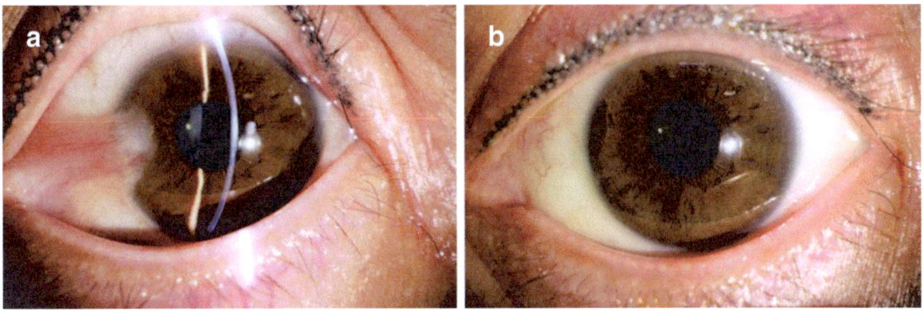

Fig. 4.3 Pterygium before and after surgery. (**a**) A 37-year-old female patient worked as an accountant. She has hereditary pterygium. She complained of cosmetic disturbance that affected her self-confidence and wanted surgery to improve her appearance. (**b**) Three weeks after improved P.E.R.F.E.C.T. surgery combined with biological amniotic membrane covering, no noticeable scar was evident on the conjunctival wound, the anastomosed paracaruncular conjunctiva, or the corneal surface. The patient was very satisfied with the surgical outcomes

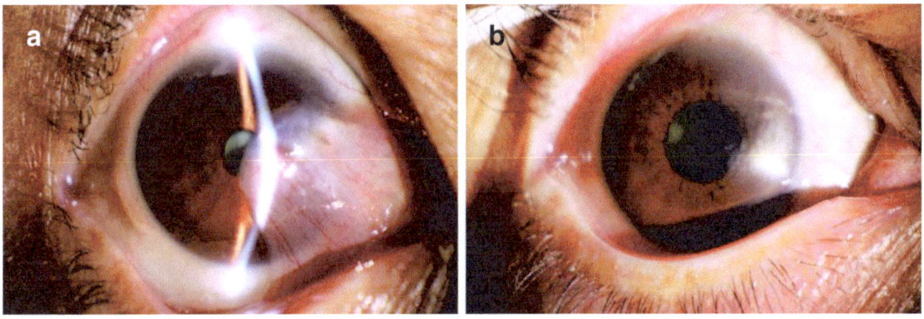

Fig. 4.4 Pterygium before and after surgery. (**a**) A 52-year-old patient was turned down at an interview because of pterygium. He sought care at our hospital and underwent surgery to improve his appearance. (**b**) One and a half years after improved P.E.R.F.E.C.T. surgery combined with biological amniotic membrane covering, the patient was very satisfied with his cosmetic appearance

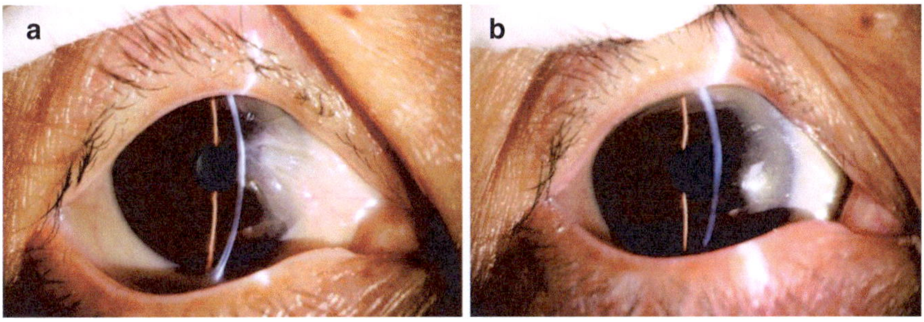

Fig. 4.5 Pterygium before and after surgery. (**a**) A 35-year-old female elementary school teacher complained that students always looked at her eye (pterygium) and thus underwent surgery to improve her appearance. (**b**) One year and 3 months after improved P.E.R.F.E.C.T. surgery combined with biological amniotic membrane covering, the patient was very satisfied

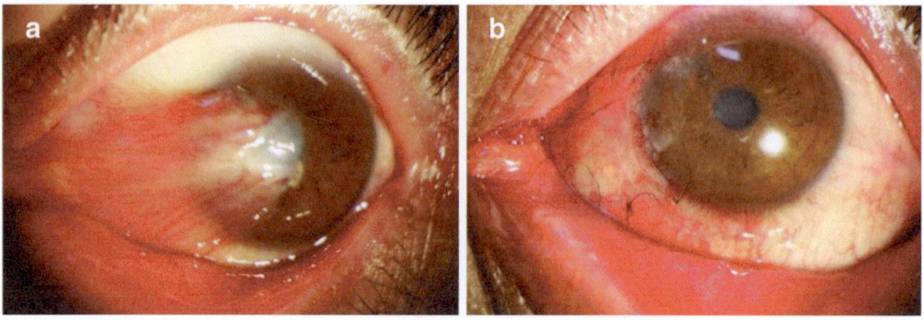

Fig. 4.6 Primary pterygium before and after surgery. (**a**) The patient had primary pterygium combined with meibomian gland dysfunction (MGD) and thus suffered mixed-type dry eye manifesting as constant eye redness and foreign body sensation. (**b**) On day 2 after improved P.E.R.F.E.C.T. surgery combined with a bandage soft contact lens covering, no signs of pterygium were noted, and the conjunctival flap remained in place. Four weeks after the surgical suture was removed, the patient was treated for dry eyes with an intense pulsed light (IPL) device featuring optimal pulse technology (OPT)

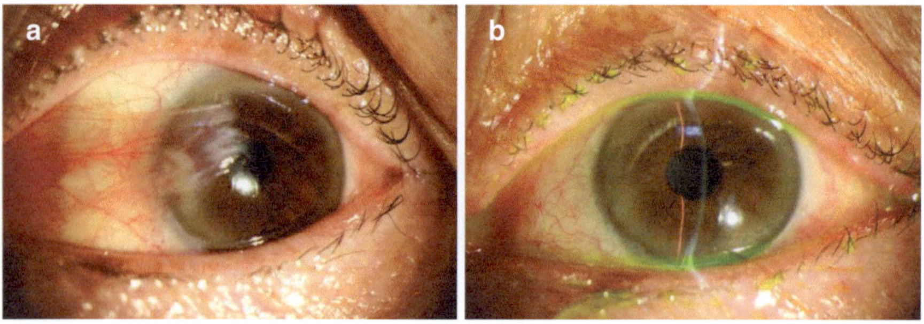

Fig. 4.7 Pterygium before and after surgery. (**a**) The patient had blurred vision in the left eye, and corneal astigmatism decreased the patient's VA to 0.3. (**b**) A half year after surgery, the patient was very satisfied with the outcome, with a visual acuity of 1.0

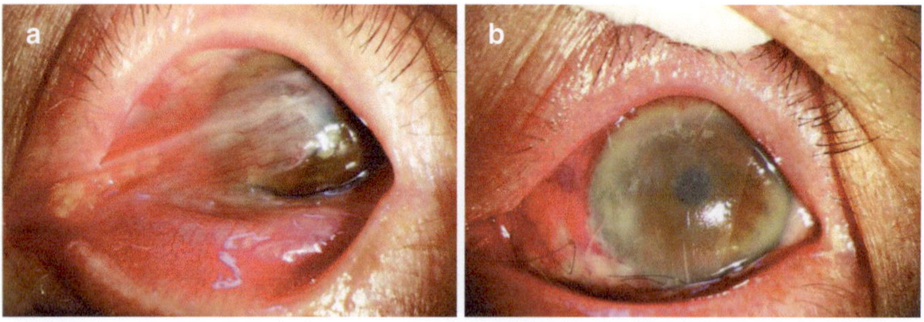

Fig. 4.8 Pterygium before and after surgery. (**a**) Affected by pterygium, this male patient was unable to roll his left eyeball outwards, had decreased vision, and often had eye redness. (**b**) One day after improved P.E.R.F.E.C.T. surgery combined with biological amniotic membrane covering, the symblepharon was released, and the amniotic membrane covering the corneal wound remained in the proper place

4.1.1.4 Precise Calculation of Corneal Curvature for Intraocular Lens (IOL) Implantation Before Cataract–IOL Surgery

Pterygium, which bulges from the corneal and conjunctival surfaces, causes dry eyes due to tear kinetic abnormalities. Moreover, the fibrovascular membrane that grows on the surface of the cornea can change the corneal curvature, and this change affects the IOL calculation for patients with cataracts. Even a small pterygium can affect accurate IOL calculation. In addition, a pterygium close to the pupil area can affect the surgeon's field of view during cataract surgery. Therefore, in patients with both pterygium and cataracts, pterygium is usually treated before cataracts (Figs. 4.9 and 4.10).

4.1.1.5 Providing a Clear Visual Pathway for Intraocular Surgery

Vitreoretinal eye surgery requires a **clear visual pathway** and transparent cornea. Pterygium passing the corneal limbus by 3 mm may affect the surgical field of vision, necessitating pterygium removal before vitreoretinal eye surgery. The principles

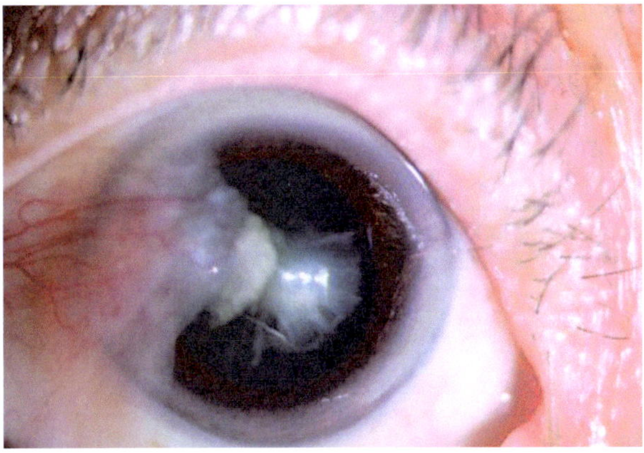

Fig. 4.9 The patient's pterygium covers the pupil optic axis and affects the measurement of the intraocular lens and the cataract surgeon's operative ability

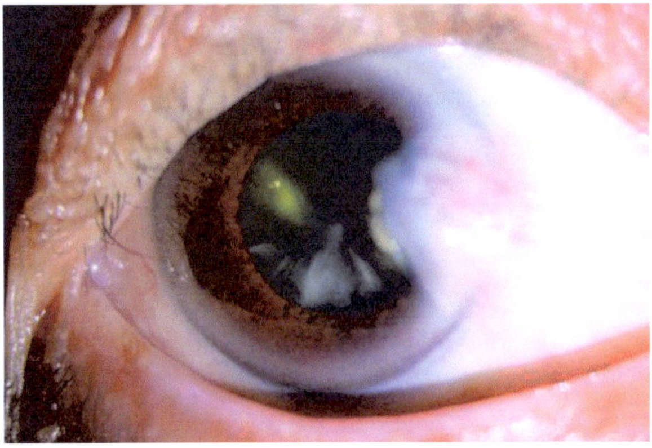

Fig. 4.10 The patient's pterygium is close to the pupil optic axis and affects the measurement of the intraocular lens and the surgeon's operative ability

regarding the relationship between pterygium treatment and surgery deep inside of the eye are as follows. First, intraocular surgery should be performed 2 weeks after pterygium surgery; these two kinds of surgeries should not be performed at the same time. Second, the success of pterygium surgery is critical because it can reduce the postoperative recurrence rate and the risk of surgical complications (Fig. 4.11).

4.1.2 Main Factors Affecting Surgical Decision-Making

4.1.2.1 Age

Primary pterygium is more common in middle-aged and elderly people, especially those over 40 years of age, and the onset of hereditary pterygium may occur at an earlier age. The onset of pterygium occurred at the ages of 4, 6, and 20 years in 3 patients of the same family [1]. The earliest pterygium onset age observed in our clinical practice was 9 years. Although no strict age limit has been imposed for pterygium surgery, surgical treatment, especially for the purpose of improving cosmetic appearance, is often performed in adult patients to reduce the risk of post-operative recurrence and complications (Fig. 4.12).

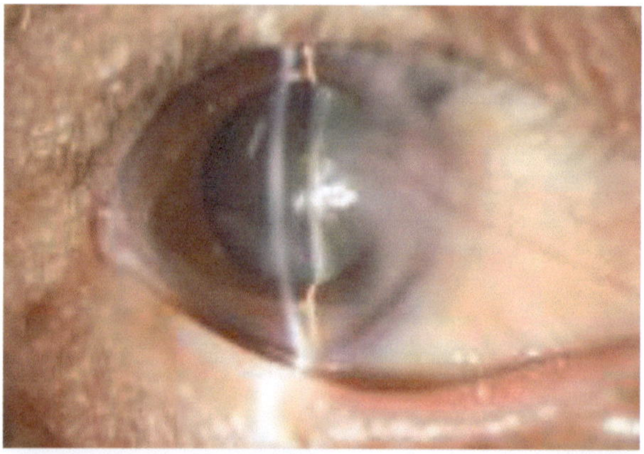

Fig. 4.11 Diabetic retinopathy and cataract complicated by primary pterygium. The patient should receive pterygium surgery first, followed by vitrectomy and cataract surgery 2 weeks later

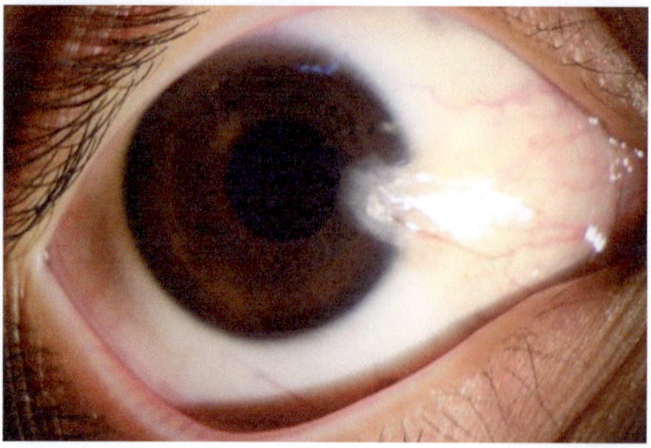

Fig. 4.12 A 9-year-old male received an initial diagnosis at our hospital, and his aunt has a similar disease, but her age of onset was 30 years old

4.1.2.2 Pterygium Size

No agreement has been reached on the pterygium size suitable for surgical treatment. Considering the high postoperative recurrence rate of pterygium, most doctors believe that surgery is unnecessary for small or regressive pterygium. However, people currently have greater cosmetic requirements with regard to their eyes because of higher living standards and a broader range of activities. Patients often seek treatment for a small pterygium or even a pinguecula that has not reached the limbus. Therefore, pterygium size is not a decisive factor for surgery; instead, surgery is often selected after a thorough discussion between the patient and the surgeon on the benefits and risks of surgery.

Surgeons should fully assess whether each patient's expectations can be met by surgery based on his/her surgical experience and skill; if not, the patient should be referred to a physician with more experience.

4.1.2.3 Timing of Surgery

Appropriate surgical timing is critical to avoid postoperative recurrence and complications. Pterygium surgery performed in patients with active inflammation might cause stronger postoperative responses and slower resolution of congestion as well as higher risks for recurrence and complications such as infection, persistent corneal epithelial defects, and inflammatory granuloma.

The timing of surgery varies with pterygium type:

1. Primary pterygium: For an advancing pterygium, surgery should be performed after inflammation is controlled. A quiescent pterygium can be surgically removed in a timely manner. For a regressive pterygium, elective surgery can be an option.
2. Recurrent pterygium:

   The second surgery should be performed at least 6 months after the first surgery and only when local inflammation is completely controlled.
3. Pseudopterygium: Pseudopterygium caused by immune diseases such as rheumatic disease should be treated initially with medications rather than surgery. Surgical treatment, when indicated, must be performed with extra caution because surgical trauma may stimulate or activate immune responses, which aggravate the primary disease and even lead to corneal dissolution/perforation. For a pseudopterygium resulting from mechanical or chemical injuries, surgery can be an option more than 1 year after injury, and the surgical approach should be determined based on the scope and depth of the lesion. Because conventional pterygium surgery will most likely not result in satisfactory outcomes, other approaches, including eye surface reconstruction, stem cell transplantation, and lamellar keratoplasty, are often performed (Figs. 3.34, 3.35, and 3.38).
4. Pterygium accompanied by blepharitis, *Demodex* mites in eyelash hair follicles, or moderate or more severe MGD must be treated first. Surgery for pte-

rygium can be an option more than 6 months after blepharitis is treated. In patients with *Demodex* mites in eyelash hair follicles, pterygium surgery should be performed after *Demodex* mites are treated for at least 3 months and a reduction in number or successful control has been confirmed. *Demodex* mites in eyelash hair follicles are reportedly one of the causes of postoperative recurrence of pterygium. In patients with simple MGD-associated dry eye, pterygium surgery can be performed either 1 month before OPT therapy or after 3 OPT treatments.

5. Dry eye: Patients with mild dry eye can undergo pterygium surgery. In patients with moderate dry eye, pterygium surgery can be performed after the patients receive anti-inflammatory treatment and corneal staining is negative. In patients with severe dry eye, the cause must be identified, and immune diseases (e.g., rheumatic disease) or connective tissue diseases should be ruled out. Pterygium surgery can be an option after patients receive systematic anti-inflammatory treatment and corneal staining is negative. In patients with extremely severe dry eye, the decision to apply pterygium surgery as a treatment approach should be made with caution.

4.2 Section 2: Indications and Contraindications for Surgery

4.2.1 Indications

1. Declining vision due to coverage of the visual axis by the pterygium;
2. Pterygium-associated recurrent inflammation leading to discomfort such as congestion in the eye, photophobia, lacrimation, and foreign body sensation;
3. Pterygium causing corneal astigmatism—In general, invasion of the corneal limbus of 3.5 mm or more by pterygium can cause corneal astigmatism of 1.0 D or higher. Astigmatism not only reduces visual acuity but also affects visual quality;
4. A need for a clear pathway inside the eye—Vitreoretinal eye surgery requires a good corneal optical surface, and IOL calculations for cataract surgery require an accurate corneal curvature. Therefore, standard pterygium surgery should be performed prior to surgery deep inside of the eye;
5. Cosmetic enhancement—Even a small pterygium can affect the cosmetic appearance of the eye. Pterygium surgery can be an option for patients who wish to improve their eye appearance;
6. Pterygium exhibiting morphological changes—Pterygium that has cyst-like changes, bleeds, or infiltrates the cornea should be surgically removed, and the excised tissue should be sent for pathological examination to confirm the diagnosis.

4.2.2 *Contraindications*

1. Eyelid abnormalities and purulent infection of the eyelid margin and appendages of the lacrimal duct, including lagophthalmos, corneal exposure, entropion with trichiasis, ulcerative blepharitis, and acute/chronic dacryocystitis;
2. Active inflammation of the eye, such as acute conjunctivitis, active trachoma, all types of keratitis or corneal ulcers, all types of uveitis, and chronic conjunctivitis with mucus discharge;
3. Recent history of allergies to medications or other agents (the surgery should be postponed);
4. Severe uncontrolled systemic disease;
5. Severe uncontrolled dry eyes;
6. Pterygium recurrence within 6 months;
7. Pseudopterygium;
8. Immune disorders (surgical decisions must be made with caution).

4.3 Section 3: Preoperative Examinations for Pterygium Surgery

4.3.1 *General Examination*

1. Blood pressure—In patients with a history of hypertension, surgery cannot be performed until blood pressure is controlled and stable. In general, before surgery, each patient should have a stable blood pressure below 160/90 mmHg.
2. Blood glucose—In patients with diabetes mellitus, preoperative fasting blood glucose should be controlled and maintained below 8.3 mmol/L.
3. Routine blood and urine tests.
4. Electrolyte testing (when necessary).
5. Four routine tests for blood transfusions.
6. Coagulation tests for patients who have taken aspirin for many years.
7. Liver and kidney function examination.
8. Electrocardiogram (ECG).
9. For patients with severe systematic disease (e.g., cerebral infarction, cerebral haemorrhage, myocardial infarction, severe arrhythmia, and sinus bradycardia), surgery must be approved by a qualified internal medical physician or anaesthesiologist who has thoroughly assessed the general conditions of the patient for surgery and documented the assessment results.
10. For patients ≥80 years old, surgery must be approved by qualified internal medicine physicians after consultation.
11. For patients with immune diseases (e.g., rheumatic disease), surgical decisions must be made with caution because uncontrolled disease may affect wound healing.

4.3.2 *Eye Examination*

1. Visual acuity and optometry.
2. Intraocular pressure (IOP) examination.
3. Routine slit-lamp anterior segment examination—Eyelids (severe entropion with trichiasis, ectropion, lagophthalmos, corneal exposure, and ulcerative blepharitis must be ruled out), pterygium (size, surface tension of the conjunctiva, and morphology of the lacrimal caruncle), cornea (all corneal thickness (CT) values and epithelial integrity/smoothness), anterior chamber depth (ACD), Tyndall phenomenon in the anterior chamber, and cells in aqueous humour.
4. Fundus examination—Patients whose visual acuity cannot be corrected and explained by the size of the pterygium and the degree of cataracts should receive further examinations for diseases of the fundus.
5. Ultrasound examination—Assessment of the axial length of the eye and the basic conditions of the retina and vitreum.
6. Lacrimal duct irrigation examination of the eye to be operated on.
7. Tear film break-up time evaluation.
8. Anterior segment imaging.
9. Corneal staining examination.
10. Anterior segment optical coherence tomography (OCT) to assess the depth of corneal scars (required for recurrent pterygium surgery).
11. Ultrasound biomicroscopy (UBM) is required when the peripheral ACD is less than 1/3 of the CT and the axial length of the eye is less than 22 mm on B ultrasound.
12. Eye movement and binocular coordination examination.

4.4 Section 4: Pterygium Assessments

4.4.1 *Grading of Primary Pterygium*

1. **Grade of primary pterygium based on the degree of corneal invasion** No universal consensus on the standards for pterygium grading has been established. Because invasion of the cornea by pterygium causes corneal astigmatism, and because the degrees of corneal invasion and corneal astigmatism are positively correlated, pterygium can be clinically graded based on the degree of corneal invasion [2, 3] (Table 4.1; Figs. 4.13, 4.14, 4.15, 4.16, and 4.17).
2. **Classification of primary pterygium based on clinical severity** Primary pterygium may be clinically categorized as mild (Grade 1), moderate (Grade 2), severe (Grade 3), and giant (Grade 4).

   The above two methods are both based on the degree of pterygium invasion into the corneal limbus without considering the degree of congestion and the protruding height of pterygium; therefore, they do not reflect the overall pterygium status.

Table 4.1 Pterygium grade based on the degree of corneal invasion

Grade	Degree of corneal invasion
Grade 0	No pterygium on the cornea
Grade 1	The pterygium head is at the limbus
Grade 2	The pterygium head is between the limbus and the pupil margin
Grade 3	The pterygium head is at the pupil margin
Grade 4	The pterygium head has passed the pupil margin

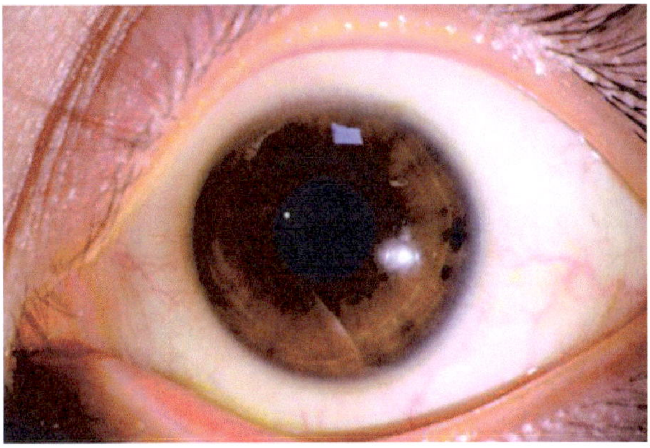

Fig. 4.13 Grade 0: no pterygium

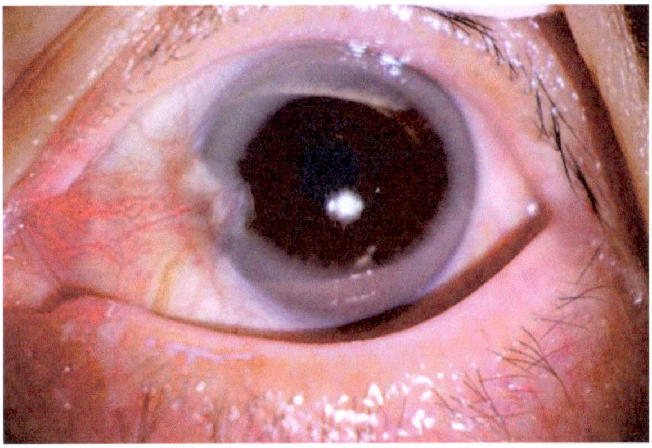

Fig. 4.14 Grade 1: the pterygium head is located at the limbus

3. **The S-V-C-K classification system** This system is applied to comprehensively assess primary pterygium in clinical research [4, 5]. S (stage) refers to the degree of corneal invasion by pterygium, V (vascularity) refers to vascular density, C (conjunctival tissue thickness) refers to the thickness of pterygium overlying the bulbar conjunctiva, and K (corneal tissue thickness) refers to the thickness of the pterygium covering the cornea (Table 4.2; Figs. 4.18, 4.19, 4.20, 4.21, and 4.22).

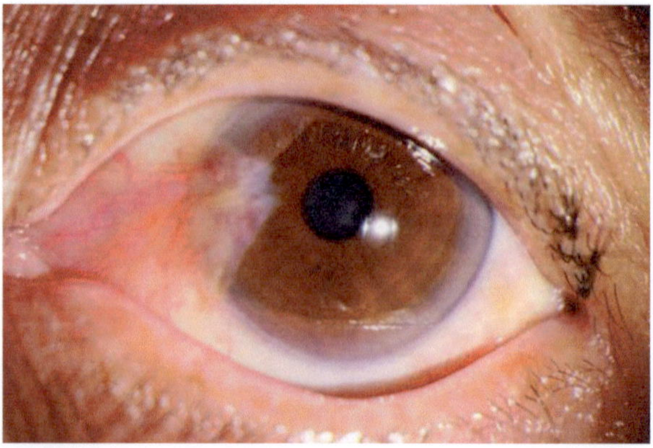

Fig. 4.15 Grade 2: the pterygium head is located between the limbus and the pupillary margin

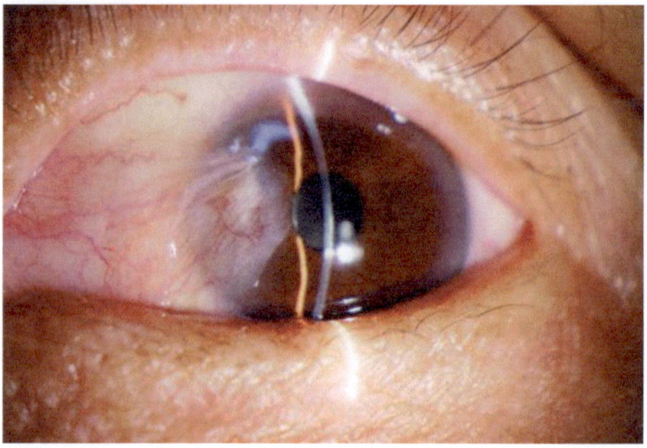

Fig. 4.16 Grade 3: the pterygium head is located at the pupillary margin

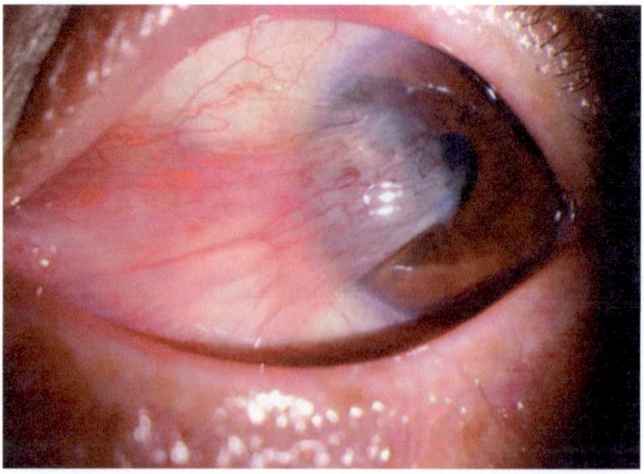

Fig. 4.17 Grade 4: the pterygium head exceeds the pupillary margin

Table 4.2 The S-V-C-K classification system for pterygium

Stage (S)
1: Pterygium invades the cornea by less than 1 mm
2: Pterygium invades the cornea by 1–2 mm
3: Pterygium invades the cornea by 2–3 mm
4: Pterygium invades the cornea more than 3 mm
Vascularity (V)
1: Pterygium has a vascular density equal to that in the conjunctiva
2: Pterygium has a vascular density higher than that in the conjunctiva
3: Pterygium has a dense vascular distribution and is congested
Conjunctival tissue thickness (C)
1: Pterygium is flat
2: Pterygium is slightly raised from the conjunctival surface
3: Pterygium is protruding from the conjunctival surface by approximately 1 mm
4: Pterygium is protruding from the conjunctival surface by more than 1 mm
Corneal tissue thickness (K)
1: Pterygium is flat
2: Pterygium is slightly elevated from the corneal surface
3: Pterygium is elevated from the corneal surface by approximately 1 mm
4: Pterygium is elevated from the corneal surface more than 1 mm

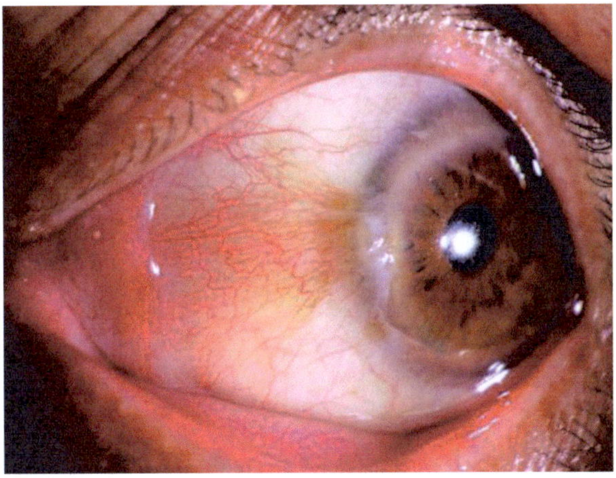

Fig. 4.18 Pterygium (S1-V1-C1-K1). The S1 pterygium head invades the corneal limbus by approximately 1 mm, the V1 vascular distribution is equivalent to that in the conjunctiva, the C1 conjunctival surface is flattened, and the K1 pterygium at corneal surface is flattened

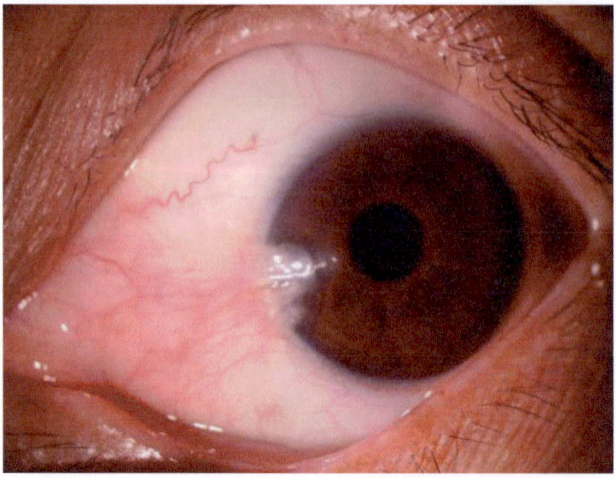

Fig. 4.19 Pterygium (S2-V1-C2-K2). The S2 pterygium head invades the corneal limbus by approximately 2 mm, the V1 vascular distribution is equivalent to that in the conjunctiva, the C2 pterygium at conjunctival surface slightly bulges by 1 mm, and the K2 pterygium at the corneal surface slightly bulges

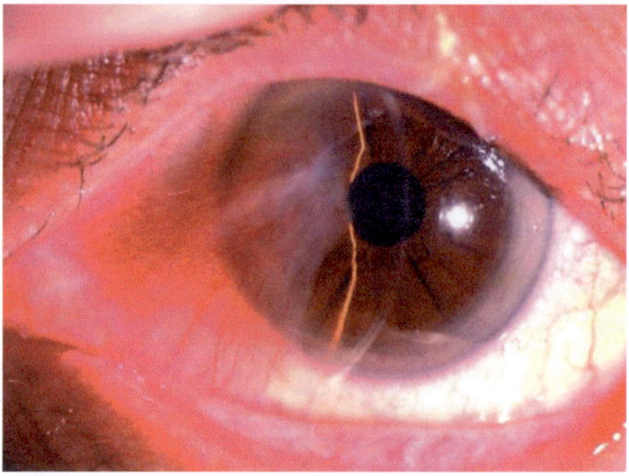

Fig. 4.20 S4 pterygium (S4-V2-C2-K1). The S4 pterygium head invades the corneal limbus by >3 mm, the V2 vascular distribution is thicker than that in the conjunctiva, the C2 pterygium at the conjunctival surface slightly bulges, and the K1 pterygium at the corneal surface is flattened

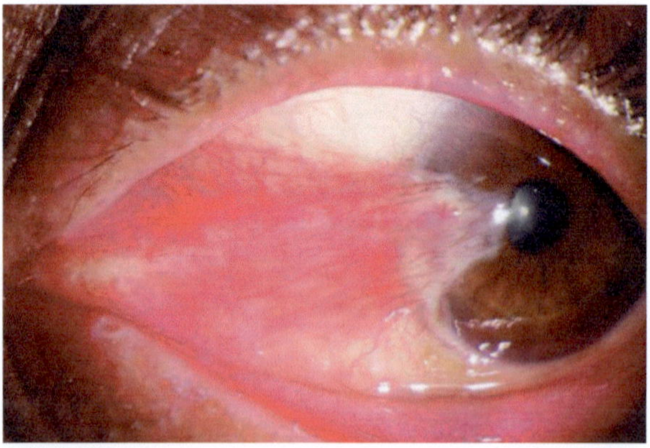

Fig. 4.21 Pterygium (S4-V2-C3-K3). The S4 pterygium head invades the corneal limbus by >3 mm, the V2 vascular distribution is thicker than that in the conjunctiva, the C3 pterygium at the conjunctival surface slightly bulges by approximately 1 mm, and the K3 pterygium at the corneal surface slightly bulges by approximately 1 mm

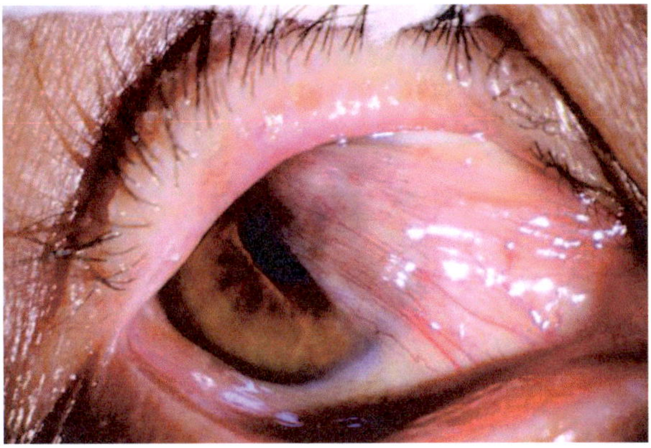

Fig. 4.22 Penicillium (S4-V1-C4-K4). The S4 pterygium head invades the cornea by >3 mm, the V1 vascular distribution is equivalent to that in the conjunctiva, the C4 pterygium at the conjunctival surface bulges by >1 mm, and the K4 pterygium at the corneal surface bulges by >1 mm

Table 4.3 Grading of the surgical area after pterygium surgery

Grade	Condition of the surgical area
Grade 1	The surgical area appears normal
Grade 2	The vessels grow to the corneal limbus, and fibrous tissue is absent
Grade 3	The fibrovascular tissue grows to the corneal limbus but has not invaded the cornea
Grade 4	The fibrovascular tissue has passed the corneal limbus and invaded the cornea

4.4.2 Outcome Assessment of Pterygium Surgery

4.4.2.1 Grading of the Surgical Area After Surgery

The grade of the surgical area after initial pterygium surgery is an important parameter for surgical outcome assessments and a major indicator used to determine pterygium recurrence. On the basis of the growth of vascular and fibrous tissues, the surgical area after initial pterygium surgery can be divided into four grades, with Grade 4 indicating pterygium recurrence [4, 6, 7] (Table 4.3; Fig. 4.23, 4.24, 4.25, and 4.26).

4.4.2.2 Cosmetic Outcome Assessments

Improving cosmetic appearance is one of the purposes of pterygium surgery. With improvements in quality of life, patients have increasingly higher requirements for satisfactory cosmetic outcomes of pterygium surgery, placing great importance on cosmetic outcome assessments. Very few existing studies have discussed the evaluation of cosmetic outcomes after pterygium surgery. Except for patients with postoperative recurrence, cosmetic outcomes are generally divided into five grades based on the condition of the conjunctival incision and morphology of the lacrimal caruncle, with Grades 1–3 considered satisfactory [7] (Table 4.4; Figs. 4.27, 4.28, 4.29, 4.30, and 4.31).

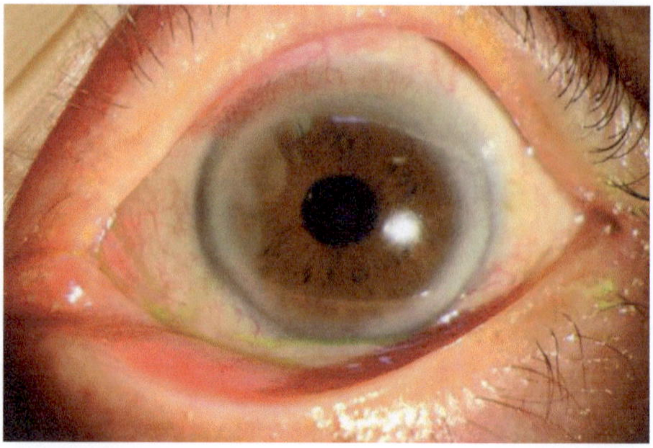

Fig. 4.23 Operative field grading after pterygium surgery, Grade 1 (normal)

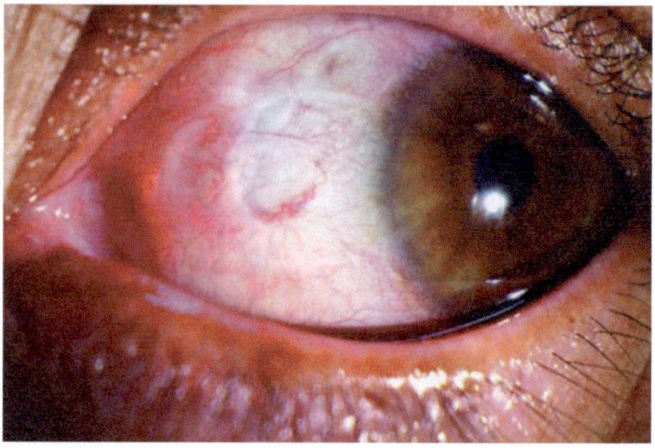

Fig. 4.24 Operative field grading after pterygium surgery, Grade 2

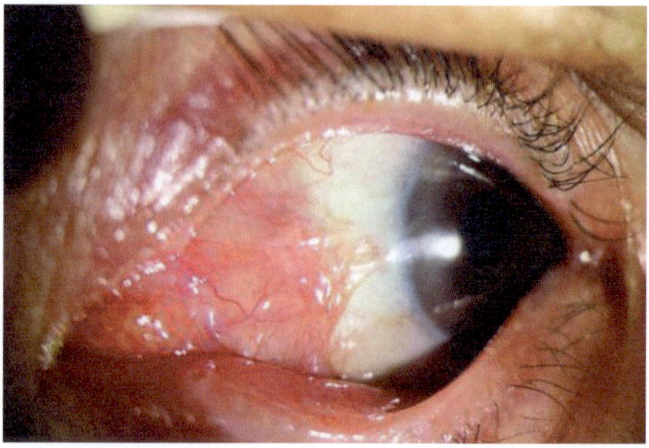

Fig. 4.25 Operative field grading after pterygium surgery, Grade 3

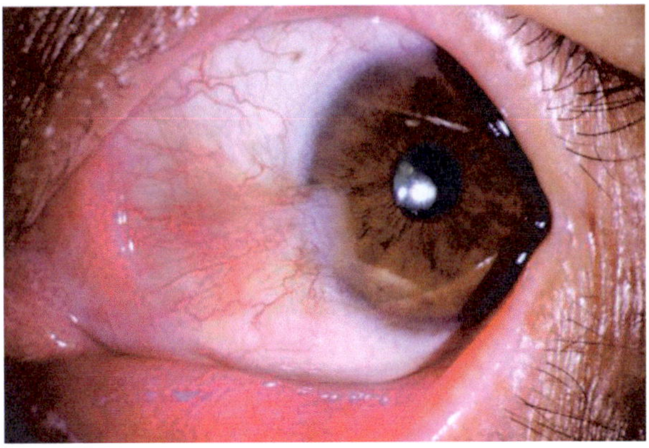

Fig. 4.26 Operative field grading after pterygium surgery, Grade 4

Table 4.4 Grading of cosmetic outcomes after pterygium surgery

Grade	Cosmetic appearance
Grade 1	The appearance is normal
Grade 2	The conjunctival incision margins have local adhesions but no thickening, and the lacrimal caruncle remains at the same position
Grade 3	The conjunctival incision margins are thickened but do not have local adhesion, and the lacrimal caruncle does not show morphological changes
Grade 4	The conjunctival incision margins have extensive adhesions, and the lacrimal caruncle has moved anteriorly by <3 mm
Grade 5	The conjunctival incision margins have extensive adhesions, and the lacrimal caruncle has moved anteriorly by >3 mm

4.4.3 Grading of Postoperative Recurrent Pterygium

Surgical techniques for pterygium have been improved by generations of ophthalmologists, such as the use of ophthalmic surgical microscopy, ophthalmic instruments, and microscopic suturing, the implementation of the conjunctival flap autografting technique, and strengthening of postoperative anti-inflammatory treatment. In conjunctival flap autografting, a healthy conjunctival flap without fascial tissue is harvested during surgery and repositioned (flat) in close contact to cover the bare scleral area, which allows a larger area of subconjunctival tissue to be excised. Although the measures above cannot completely prevent pterygium recurrence, compared to surgery performed under direct vision, microscopic surgery significantly reduces the severity and simplifies the treatment of recurrent pterygium.

On the basis of the position of recurrent pterygium and whether it is accompanied by symblepharon, pterygium recurrence can be divided into three levels: mild, moderate, and severe (Table 4.5; Figs. 4.32, 4.33, and 4.34).

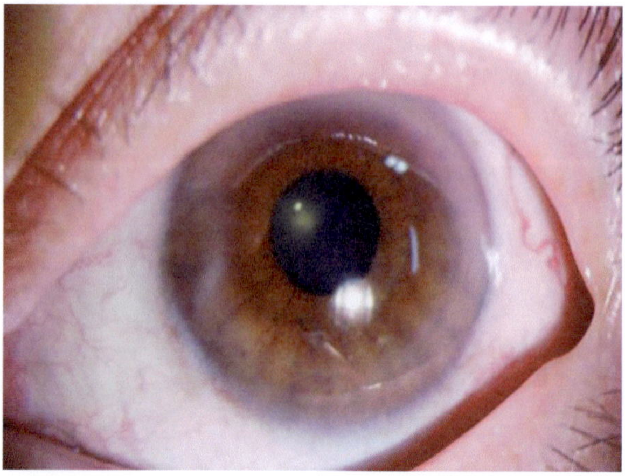

Fig. 4.27 Aesthetic effect grading after pterygium surgery, Grade 1: normal appearance

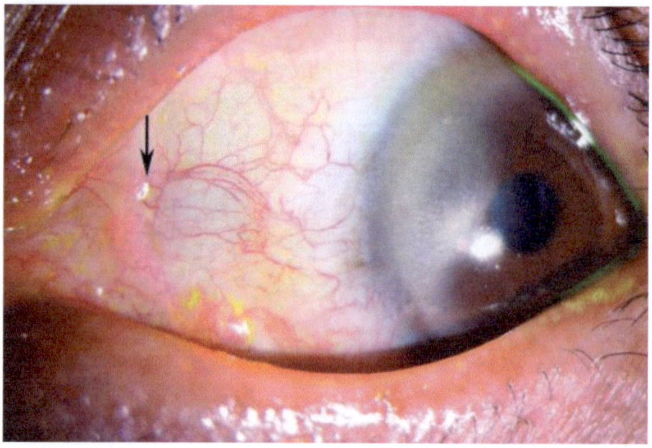

Fig. 4.28 Aesthetic effect grading after pterygium surgery, Grade 2: focal adhesions at the edge of the conjunctival incision but no thickening at the edge of the conjunctival incision or change in the position of the lacrimal caruncle (indicated by the black arrow)

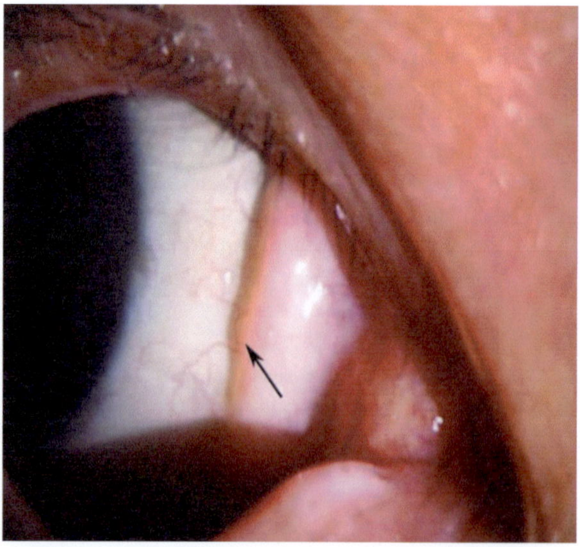

Fig. 4.29 Aesthetic effect grading after pterygium surgery, Grade 3: thickening at the edge of the conjunctival incision (indicated by the black arrow) but no obvious adhesion or morphological change in the lacrimal caruncle

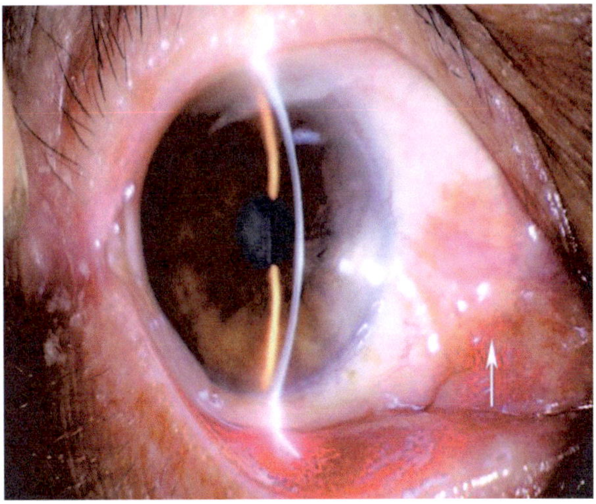

Fig. 4.30 Aesthetic effect grading after pterygium surgery, Grade 4: wide adhesion at the edge of the conjunctival incision (indicated by the white arrow), and the lacrimal caruncle shows antidisplacement by <3 mm

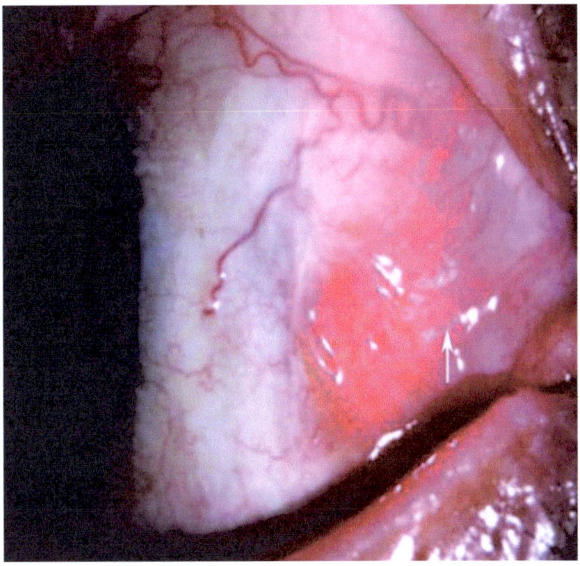

Fig. 4.31 Aesthetic effect grading after pterygium surgery, Grade 5: wide adhesion at the edge of the conjunctival incision (indicated by the white arrow), and the lacrimal caruncle shows antidisplacement by >3 mm

Table 4.5 Levels of pterygium recurrence severity

Level	Appearance
Mild	Recurrent pterygium invades the corneal limbus by less than 1 mm
Moderate	Recurrent pterygium invades the corneal limbus by 1–3 mm, without symblepharon
Severe	Recurrent pterygium invades the corneal limbus by more than 3 mm, with symblepharon

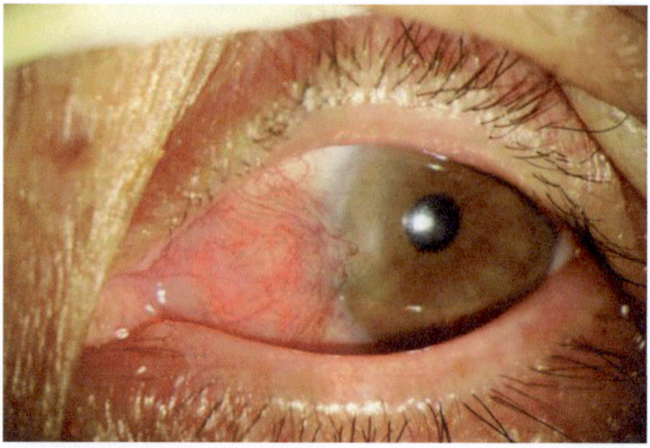

Fig. 4.32 Mild recurrence: recurrent pterygium <1 mm within the corneal limbus

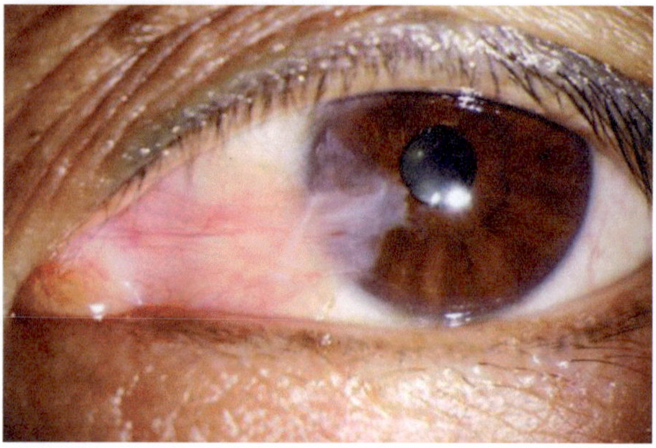

Fig. 4.33 Moderate recurrence: recurrent pterygium 1–3 mm within the corneal limbus, without symblepharon

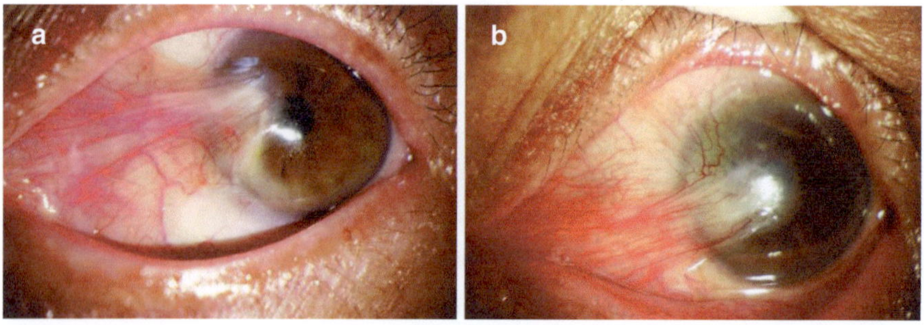

Fig. 4.34 Severe pterygium recurrence. (**a**, **b**) Recurrent pterygium invaded the corneal limbus by more than 3 mm, with symblepharon

Key Points

Currently, pterygium surgery is still performed under direct vision in some primary hospitals in China, potentially leading to significantly stronger postoperative responses, severe wound pain, and a higher postoperative recurrence rate. We suggest that more effort should be made to promote microscopic surgery (Figs. 4.35, 4.36, 4.37, 4.38, and 4.39).

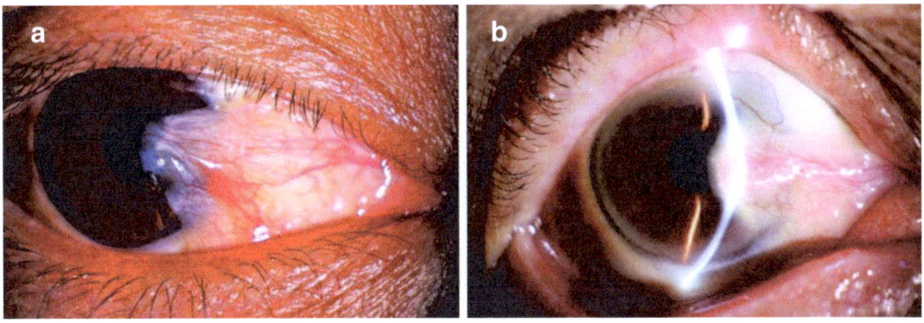

Fig. 4.35 Recurrence after pterygium microsurgery. (**a**, **b**) The recurrent lesion is still in the superficial layer of the corneal stroma, without obvious symblepharon

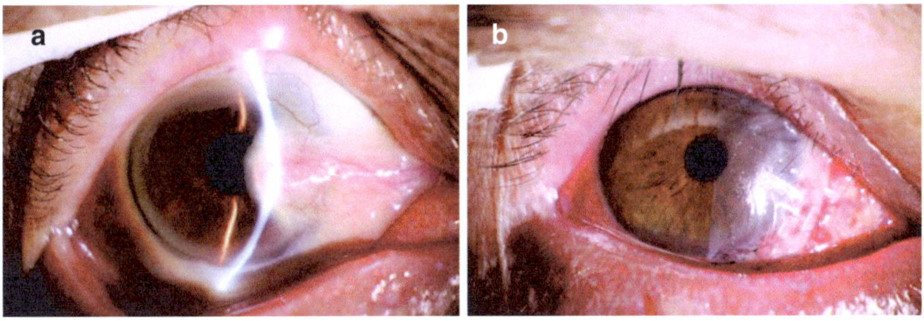

Fig. 4.36 Recurrence after pterygium microsurgery, before and after secondary surgery. (**a**) Before surgery: the recurrent lesion is still in the superficial layer of the corneal stroma, without obvious symblepharon. (**b**) The patient needs only modified P.E.R.F.E.C.T. plus biological amniotic membrane covering; the appearance on the second postoperative day

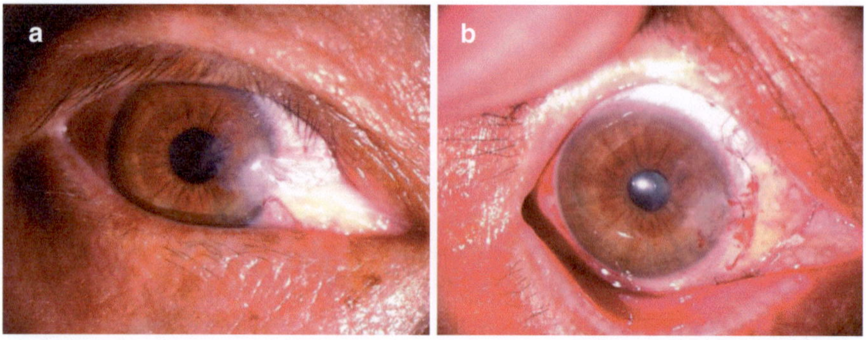

Fig. 4.37 Recurrence after pterygium nonmicrosurgery, before and after secondary surgery. (**a**) A patient with recurrence after nonmicrosurgery for pterygium showing severe symblepharon, the eyeball fixed on the nasal side, a visual acuity of 0.6, and no invasion at the pupil area who received conjunctival flap transplantation with stem cells. (**b**) Recurrent pterygium resection + symblepharon dissociation + conjunctival flap transplantation with stem cells in the patient's right eye; visual acuity was restored to 1.0 upon suture removal on the seventh postoperative day

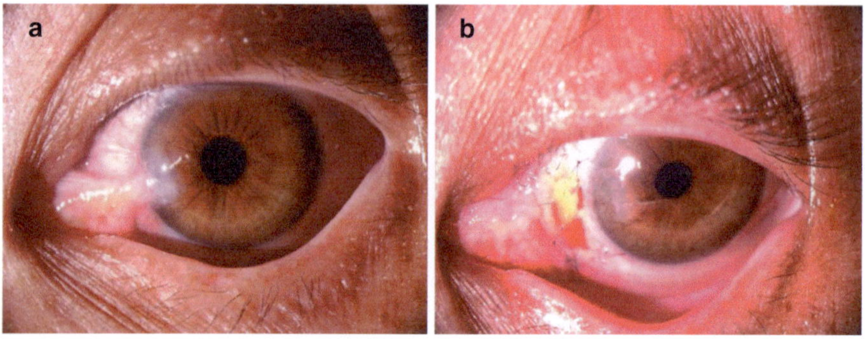

Fig. 4.38 Recurrence after pterygium nonmicrosurgery, before and after secondary surgery. (**a**) The same patient in Fig. 4.37: his or her left eye developed recurrence after nonmicrosurgery for pterygium, with severe symblepharon, the eyeball fixed on the nasal side, a visual acuity of 0.8, and no invasion at the pupil area, and the patient received conjunctival flap transplantation with stem cells; (**b**) recurrent pterygium resection + symblepharon dissociation + conjunctival flap transplantation with stem cells in the patient's left eye; visual acuity was restored to 1.2 upon suture removal on the seventh postoperative day

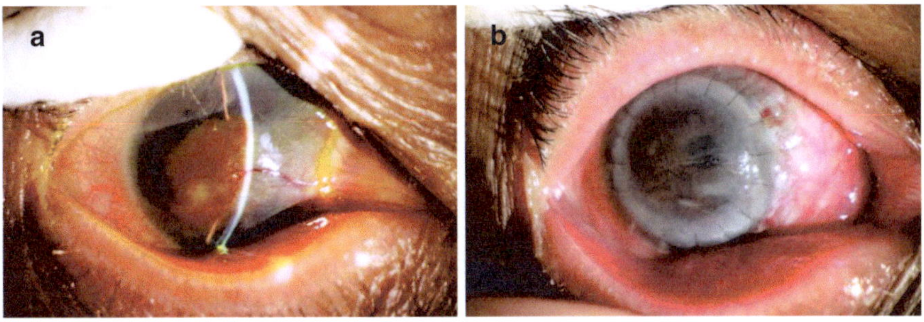

Fig. 4.39 Recurrence after pterygium nonmicrosurgery, before and after secondary surgery. (**a**) A patient with recurrence after nonmicrosurgery for pterygium showing severe symblepharon, the eyeball fixed on the nasal side, corneal stromal scarring, neovascularization into the corneal stroma, vascular rupture and bleeding, and a visual acuity of "hand movement". (**b**) At 2 weeks after lamellar keratoplasty, symblepharon was relieved, eye movement was free, and visual acuity was restored to 0.08

References

1. Islam SI, Wagoner MD. Pterygium in young member of one family. Cornea. 2001;20:708–10.
2. Tan CSH, Lim TH, Koh WP, et al. Epidemiology of pterygium on a tropical island in the Riau Archipelago. Eye (Lond). 2006;20(8):908–12.
3. Zhong H, Cha X, Wei T, et al. Prevalence of and risk factors for pterygium in rural adult Chinese populations of the Bai nationality in Dali: the Yunnan Minority Eye Study. Invest Ophthalmol Vis Sci. 2012;53(10):6617–21.
4. Kim DJ, Lee JK, Chuck RS, et al. Low recurrence rate of anchored conjunctival rotation flap technique in pterygium surgery. BMC Ophthalmol. 2017;17(1):187.
5. Park CY, Choi JS, Lee SJ, et al. Cyclooxygenase-2-expressing macrophages in human pterygium co-express vascular endothelial growth factor. Mol Vis. 2011;17:3468–80.
6. Prabhasawat P, Barton K, Burkett G, et al. Comparison of conjunctival autografts, amniotic membrane grafts, and primary closure for pterygium excision. Ophthalmology. 1997;104(6):974–85.
7. Liu HY, Chen YF, Chen TC, et al. Surgical result of pterygium extended removal followed by fibrin glue-assisted amniotic membrane transplantation. J Formos Med Assoc. 2017;116(1):10–7.

Chapter 5
Perioperative Management of Pterygium

Congxiang Wang

5.1 Section 1: Management of Related Diseases

5.1.1 Management of the Local Eye Environment

5.1.1.1 Treatment of Eyelid Disease

Lagophthalmos affects corneal wound healing and may also cause exposure keratitis or other corneal infections, especially in patients with poor Bell's phenomenon. Hence, lagophthalmos must be managed prior to pterygium surgery. Patients with lagophthalmos should be transferred to a plastic surgery department for treatment and should not undergo pterygium surgery until their eyelids can completely close. Infectious eyelid diseases, including blepharitis, meibomian gland cyst infection, and eyelid skin purulent diseases, should be properly treated and controlled before pterygium surgery (Fig. 5.1).

5.1.1.2 Eyelid Margin and Ocular Surface Conditions

Attention must be directed towards managing the conditions of the eyelid margin and ocular surface prior to pterygium surgery. Anterior blepharitis is often accompanied by staphylococcal infection or seborrheic dermatitis, which can lead to massive bacterial growth on the corneal wound surface and increase the risk of infection after pterygium surgery. Posterior blepharitis is mostly caused by MGD. Mild posterior blepharitis can lead to dry eyes associated with lipid abnormalities, and severe posterior blepharitis can cause blepharokerato conjunctivitis (BKC). Patients should receive a corneal staining examination prior to pterygium surgery. A stained cornea,

C. Wang (✉)
Changsha Aier Eye Hospital, Changsha, China

C. Wang, S. Li (eds.), *Pterygium Surgery*,
https://doi.org/10.1007/978-981-99-6843-5_5

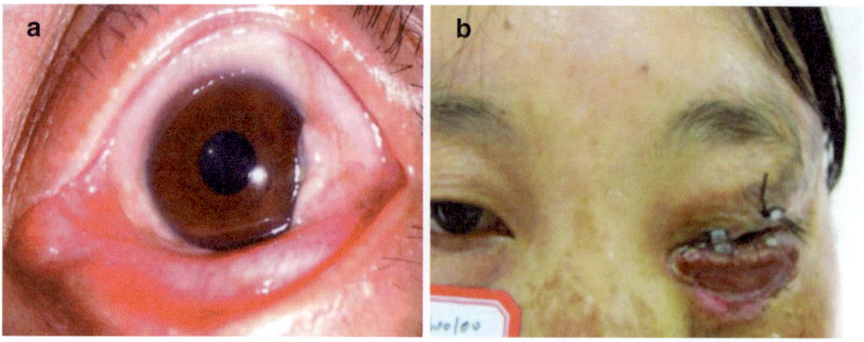

Fig. 5.1 Primary pterygium combined with cicatricial ectropion of the lower eyelid. (**a**) Pterygium combined with cicatricial ectropion of the lower eyelid. (**b**) The patient was transferred to the plastic surgery department and treated to correct lower eyelid cicatricial ectropion and then underwent pterygium surgery

an obvious skin ulcer on the eyelid margin, and pustular/papules or cuff-like secretions at the root of the eyelashes, as well as corneal infiltration and neovascularization in the interpalpebral area, may indicate BKC. Pterygium surgery must be postponed until blepharitis is cured.

5.1.1.3 Treatment of Chronic Dacryocystitis

Chronic dacryocystitis is an absolute contraindication to pterygium surgery and must be treated seriously. Modern lacrimal duct surgery is mostly minimally invasive and is easy and simple, with a quick patient recovery; postoperative lacrimal duct irrigation should be administered to ensure the patency of the new lacrimal duct system before pterygium surgery.

5.1.1.4 Management of a Shallow Anterior Chamber

In an eye with a shallow anterior chamber, surgery may result in acute angle-closure glaucoma. To manage a shallow anterior chamber in patients with small eyeballs, a short eye axis, or hyperopia, special attention should be given to the opening of the chamber angle. When the peripheral ACD is less than 1/4 of the CT, a UBM examination should be performed to determine the presence of chamber angle closure. Patients with a chamber angle closure greater than 1/2 should be transferred to the glaucoma department for YAG laser iridotomy, followed by pterygium surgery 1 week later. Without properly treating a shallow anterior chamber, epinephrine-free anaesthetics are insufficient to prevent acute angle-closure glaucoma because it may be triggered by pupil dilation associated with surgical stimulation and eye bandaging (Fig. 5.2).

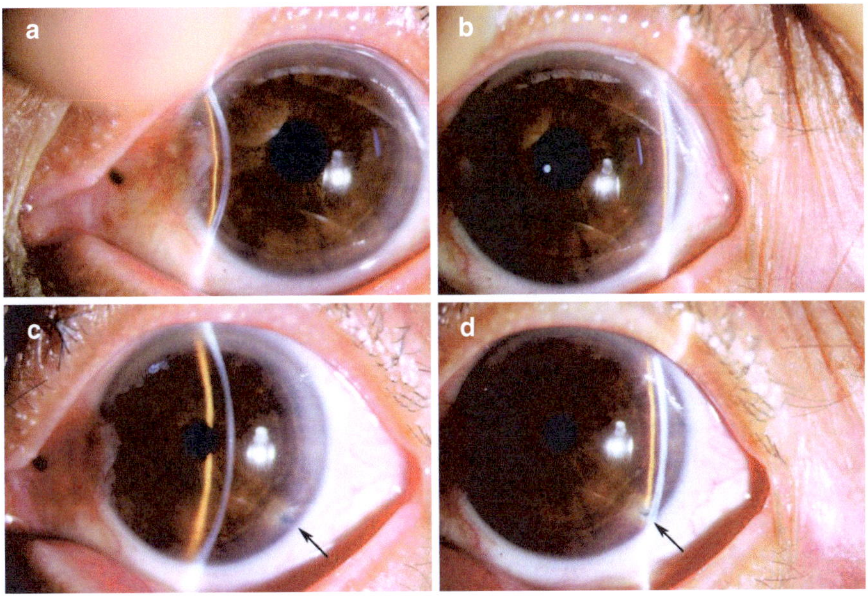

Fig. 5.2 The patient had a shallow anterior chamber and an eye axis length of 21.5 mm; UBM revealed narrowing and partial closure of the chamber angle. (**a**) The mid-periphery ACD (nasal side) was approximately 1 mm. (**b**) The peripheral ACD was approximately 1/4 of the CT. After communication and discussion, the patient understood and agreed with the treatment plan that pterygium surgery would be performed after YAG laser iridotomy. (**c**) After Nd:YAG laser surgery, the central anterior chamber became deeper (the black arrow denotes the laser hole). (**d**) The peripheral ACD was 1 mm, and the laser hole was open (black arrow), allowing pterygium surgery to be performed 7 days later

5.1.1.5 Management of Fundus Complications in High Myopia

Common fundus complications of high myopia include dry holes and lattice degeneration of the peripheral retina, rhegmatogenous retinal detachment, and macular haemorrhage. Before pterygium surgery, patients with high myopia should receive treatment to correct their vision and should be given a thorough fundus examination (ultrawide-field fundus photography or consultation with a retinal specialist if necessary) to rule out fundus diseases. Dry hole and lattice degeneration of the retina should be treated with fundus laser therapy to close the hole prior to pterygium surgery. Retinal detachment and macular haemorrhage should be managed following the advice of the retina specialist. For patients with the abovementioned diseases, the doctor must explain the causes and prognosis to the patient in detail and perform pterygium surgery only after he or she understands and agrees with the treatment plan.

5.1.2 Management of Systemic Conditions

Blood pressure, blood glucose, and routine general examinations and requirements are described in Sect. 4.3 of Chap. 4. Pterygium surgery is an elective surgery requiring a full consultation with a specialist or anaesthesiologist to ensure the safety of patients with cardiovascular and cerebrovascular diseases. Surgery can be performed only when the conditions below have been well controlled [1].

1. **Sinus bradycardia:** If a patient has a heart rate less than 50 beats per minute, an atropine injection and 24-h Holter electrocardiogram should be administered to measure the slowest heart rate and its duration. If the heart rate does not increase after an atropine injection, pterygium surgery should be postponed until the patient has been treated by a cardiologist.
2. **Sinus tachycardia:** Surgery generally requires a heart rate in the range of 60–100 beats per minute. For a patient with a heart rate exceeding 110 beats per minute, surgery can be performed only after evaluation and treatment by a cardiologist.
3. **Arrhythmia:** Patients with simple sinus arrhythmias or premature atrial contractions can receive surgery under the monitoring of an anaesthesiologist. Patients with frequent ventricular premature beats, bigeminy, trigeminy, or multifocal premature beats cannot undergo surgery and should be transferred to the cardiology department. They can receive surgical treatment for pterygium after their heart condition stabilizes.
4. **Atrial fibrillation:** The heart rate of patients with atrial fibrillation should be controlled at 60–100 beats per minute for surgery. When the heart rate of a pterygium patient is higher than 100 beats per minute, the surgeon must consult with a cardiologist and treat the patient appropriately before surgery.
5. **Ventricular fibrillation:** This is an absolute contraindication.
6. **Myocardial infarction:** Patients with an old inferior wall myocardial infarction or anterior/posterior myocardial infarction can undergo pterygium surgery. However, extensive myocardial infarction or myocardial infarction within 3 months must be treated by cardiologists before a surgical decision can be made.
7. **Atrioventricular (AV) block:** Patients with a first-degree type 1 AV block can undergo surgery. Second-degree type 2 and third-degree type 1 AV blocks should be treated before surgery. Patients with a complete right bundle branch block can undergo surgery under the monitoring of an anaesthesiologist. For patients with a complete left bundle branch block who have symptoms, surgery can be performed after treatment or when indicated by an anaesthesiologist.
8. **Cerebral infarction:** Pterygium surgery can be performed 6 months following cerebral infarction.
9. **Cerebral haemorrhage:** Pterygium surgery can be performed 6 months following cerebral **haemorrhage**.

5.2 Section 2: Perioperative Medication

The perioperative period is defined as 3 days before surgery to 1 month after surgery in the *Chinese Expert Consensus on Perioperative Medication in Pterygium Surgery (2017)* [2]. The *Standardized Treatment for Pterygium* written by Professors Jin Yuan, Jing Hong, and Xiaoming Yan and reviewed/edited by Professors Lixin Xie and Zuguo Liu states that "the perioperative period of pterygium surgery includes the entire process of preoperative preparation, surgery, and postoperative recovery until the corneal and conjunctival wound heals and ocular surface inflammation has essentially subsided; hence, the perioperative period is from 3 days before surgery to 3 months after surgery."

Perioperative medications for pterygium include the following three categories [3]:

1. Antibiotics: Antibiotics are used to prevent corneal wound infections. The antibiotics used perioperatively must have low resistance, a broad spectrum, and high efficacy. Corneal wound infection is a catastrophic event that may cause corneal clouds or white spots in mild cases and may require keratoplasty in severe cases, resulting in irreparable losses to patients. Most pterygium patients are from rural areas and have varying degrees of inflammation in the eyelid margin and the ocular surface. Special attention should be given to the conditioned pathogens in the eyelid margin. Therefore, effective broad-spectrum antibiotics must be chosen and appropriately used prior to surgery.
2. Anti-inflammatory drugs: High-efficacy, short-term anti-inflammatory treatment should be administered to patients before and after pterygium surgery to control inflammation in a timely manner. This approach accelerates the repair of the corneal epithelium and reduces the risk of recurrence, thereby minimizing patient suffering.
3. Artificial tears: Dry eyes are a common problem after pterygium surgery. Regular replenishment of artificial tears facilitates tear film recovery.

5.2.1 Preoperative Medication

1. **Antibiotics:** Gatifloxacin eye gel is applied 3 times/day, tobramycin eye drops are applied 4 times/day, or 0.5% levofloxacin eye drops are applied 4 times/day 3 days before surgery for prophylactic purposes. One day before surgery, antibiotics are applied once an hour for 12 h.
2. **Anti-inflammatory drugs:** Tobramycin-dexamethasone eye drops are applied twice a day 2 days before surgery and 3 times per day 1 day before surgery.

   Pterygium surgery is a nonemergency procedure, and successful inflammation management before surgery can reduce the risk of recurrence and postoperative responses. Advanced pterygium can be treated using tobramycin-dexamethasone eye drops (3 times a day for 3 days); if congestion remains, surgery should be postponed until inflammation is controlled.

3. **Artificial tears:** All pterygium patients have varying degrees of dry eyes. Preoperative use of artificial tears alleviates dry eye symptoms, lubricates the ocular surface, reduces the postoperative inflammatory response, and promotes epithelial repair.

5.2.2 Intraoperative Medication [4]

1. **Anaesthetics** For surface anaesthesia, oxybuprocaine hydrochloride or proparacaine hydrochloride eye drops are applied 3 times at 3-min intervals. For subconjunctival infiltration anaesthesia, a mixture of 2 mL of 0.1% lidocaine and 0.05 mL of 0.1% epinephrine hydrochloride should be applied.
2. **Drug administration in the conjunctiva sac** After surgery, tobramycin-dexamethasone eye ointment can be administered to the conjunctival sac. The operated eye is then covered with gauze and bandaged. After 2–12 h, the bandage should be opened to apply eye drops. An eye bandage can promote corneal epithelial repair, secure the implanted conjunctival flap, and relieve wound pain.

5.2.3 Postoperative Medication

The purpose of postoperative medication is to prevent infection, reduce inflammation, relieve wound pain, and promote epithelial repair.

1. **Antibiotics** Gatifloxacin eye gel is applied 3 times/day, tobramycin eye drops are applied 4 times/day, or 0.5% levofloxacin eye drops are applied 4 times/day for a total of 7–10 days.
2. **Anti-inflammatory drugs:** Tobramycin-dexamethasone eye drops are applied 4 times/day in the first week and reduced by 1 application 1 day each week thereafter for 4 weeks.
3. **Artificial tears:** Eye drops containing deproteinized calf blood extract, with the dual effects of accelerating epithelial repair and serving as artificial tears, are applied 4 times a day for 7 days. After epithelial repair, regular artificial tears, such as sodium hyaluronate and polyvinyl alcohol artificial tears, can be used. Artificial tears may be used either as needed or continuously for 3 months based on the eye condition.

5.2.4 *Surgical Wound Management*

After surgical removal of pterygium, corneal and conjunctival wounds can be managed using either of the two methods below:

1. Bandage contact lens—The patient can wear a bandage contact lens to cover the corneal wound surface after surgery; and
2. Biological amniotic membrane—The corneal and conjunctival wound surface can be covered by multiple layers of the amniotic membrane (see the related chapters/sections for details).

References

1. Zhang SY. Perioperative management of cardiovascular diseases. Beijing: People's Medical Publishing House; 2014.
2. Chinese Branch of the Asian Dry Eye Society. Chinese expert consensus on perioperative medication in pterygium surgery. Chin J Ophthalmol. 2017;53(9):653–6.
3. Liu ZG, Chen JQ. Ocular surface diseases. Beijing: People's Medical Publishing House; 2003.
4. Shi WY, Wang FH. Mitomycin C-related complications should not be neglected in pterygium surgery. Chin J Ophthalmol. 2013;49(10):869–72.

Chapter 6
Primary Pterygium Surgery

Congxiang Wang

Surgery is the only effective treatment for pterygium. Common surgical procedures for pterygium in clinical practice at home and abroad include simple pterygium excision, pterygium excision with bioamnion transplantation, pterygium excision with free conjunctival flap autograft, pterygium excision with limbal stem cell transplantation, etc. Although the latter two procedures are most widely used, they are still associated with a certain recurrence rate and less than satisfactory in terms of aesthetics and postoperative pain [1].

The essential measures to reduce the postoperative recurrence rate of pterygium are as follows: (1) operation by experienced surgeons; (2) radical excision of pterygium; (3) determination of the optimal surgical procedure according to the size, growth pattern and inflammation severity of pterygium; (4) strict perioperative medication. After decades of investigation on pterygium surgery at home and abroad, the author invented six surgical procedures with reference to the existing advantages, of which the modified Perfect not only has no recurrence and few complications, but also produces excellent aesthetic results. Moreover, the combination with bioamnion covering can alleviate postoperative xerophthalmia, accelerate the healing of corneal and conjunctival epithelium and increase ocular comfort of patients. The six surgical procedures for primary pterygium commonly used in the author's hospital are introduced as follows.

Supplementary Information The online version contains supplementary material available at https://doi.org/10.1007/978-981-99-6843-5_6.

C. Wang (✉)
Changsha Aier Eye Hospital, Changsha, China

C. Wang, S. Li (eds.), *Pterygium Surgery*,
https://doi.org/10.1007/978-981-99-6843-5_6

6.1 Part I: Conventional Pterygium Excision with Free Conjunctival Flap Autograft

6.1.1 Indications

1. Primary pterygium.
2. More effective in the following cases:

   (a) Horizontally growing pterygium with <3 mm invasion of corneal limbus;
   (b) Static pterygium;
   (c) Pterygium in patients over 70 years of age requiring cataract surgery.

6.1.2 Surgical Steps

1. Anesthesia: Topical anesthesia with subconjunctival local infiltration anesthesia is usually used in pterygium surgery; general anesthesia is also a choice for those with high mental stress and obstacles to cooperation. On the premise that the shallow anterior chamber has been treated, 1 drop of 1% epinephrine can be added to anesthetic agents for local infiltration to reduce intraoperative bleeding. During infiltration anesthesia, insert the syringe with its needle obliqually downward, inject the 0.5–1.0 mL anesthetic from the depth of 3 mm below the bulbar conjunctiva at the pterygium neck, and squeeze bulbar conjunctiva with a cotton swab or absorbent sponge soaked with normal saline to help spread anesthetic, while achieving anesthetic and analgesic effects, and separating the bulbar conjunctiva from fascia (Figs. 6.1 and 6.2).
2. Eyeball fixation: Suture the sclera at 1/2 depth by traction with 5-0 nylon suture from the corneoscleral margin at 6 o'clock, and draw the eyeball to the contralateral side of the lesion and fix it to fully expose the surgical area (Fig. 6.3).
3. Incision making and separation of bulbar conjunctiva for excision of pterygium: Radical excision of pterygium is the key to prevent recurrence. According to the common practice of conventional pterygium excision, take the terminus of

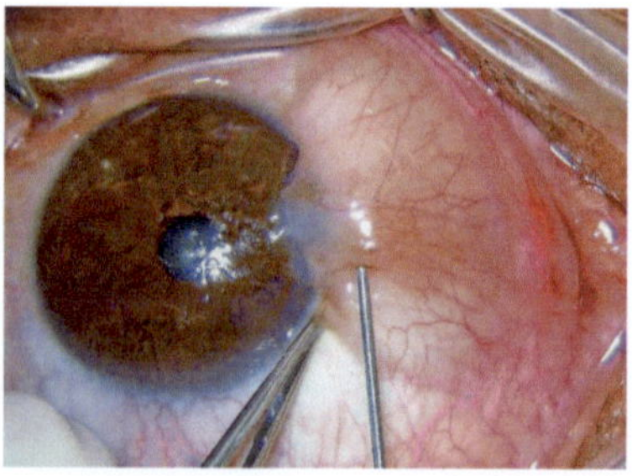

Fig. 6.1 Intraoperative anesthesia for pterygium. The needle was inserted 3 mm under the conjunctiva of the neck of the pterygium, and 0.5–1.0 ml anesthetic was injected

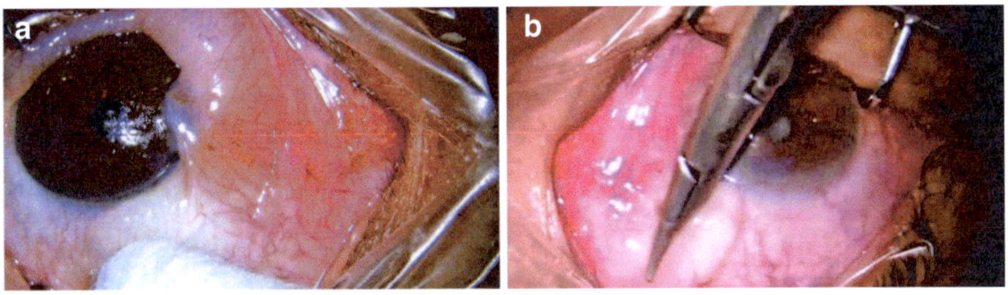

Fig. 6.2 Squeeze bulbar conjunctiva with a cotton swab or absorbent sponge soaked with normal saline to help spread anesthetic. (**a**) Cotton swabs soaked with normal saline; (**b**) squeeze bulbar conjunctiva with a microneedle holder to help spread anesthetic

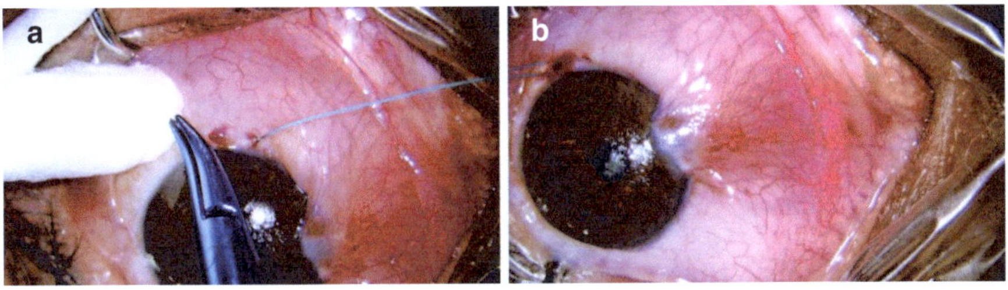

Fig. 6.3 Fixation of eyeballs. (**a**) Suture the sclera by traction with 5-0 nylon suture from the corneoscleral margin; (**b**) fully expose the surgical area

medial rectus 5.5 mm from the corneal limbus as the resection range. For beginners, first measure the distance with a gauge and then draw a conjunctival incision line with a marker. Sever it to the terminus of medial rectus along the upper and lower margins of pterygium until it reaches the terminus of medial rectus, disassociate the bulbar conjunctiva on the pterygium surface at the terminus of medial rectus parallel to the corneal limbus, and make an incision on the bulbar conjunctiva only without hurting the surrounding tissue.

Lift the conjunctiva at the upper, lower, and nasal bulbar conjunctival incisions in sequence, and bluntly exfoliate the fascia at 1 mm above and below the incisions and 2 mm from the terminus of medial rectus. Disassociate the bulbar conjunctiva and fascia under the conjunctival incision with closed microscissors and cut it open by about 3 mm with the blades. Radical dissection of fascia adjacent to pterygium by effective separation of the bulbar conjunctiva from its inferior fascia is a key step to reduce recurrence of postoperative pterygium. Besides, separate the fascia at the pterygium body from the sclera, even if no adhesion is found between the primary pterygium and its inferior sclera, after disconnecting the bulbar conjunctiva and the fascia, for the purposes of minimizing the residual fascia in the surgical area on the scleral surface and protecting the blood vessels; perform a blunt dissection and sever the upper and lower fascia after that.

Make a scratch on the pterygium head along the corneal surface to the depth of corneal epithelial layer with closed ophthalmic microscissors, clamp the pterygium head with a toothed forceps, and then exfoliate it along the corneal surface to the neck with microscissors. Next, clamp the pterygium head with a toothed forceps again, and bluntly exfoliate the neck of pterygium with closed microscissors until the pterygium is completely dissociated from the corneal surface and limbus, at which time, its three surfaces have been completely disassociated.

Clamp the head of pterygium horizontally with a toothed forceps and pull it towards the cornea for full exposure under a certain tension, and excise the pterygium at the terminus of medial rectus with microscissors (Figs. 6.4, 6.5, 6.6, 6.7, 6.8, and 6.9).

4. Wound hemostasis: During the surgical procedures for pterygium, sterilized cotton balls are usually torn and temporarily twisted into small cotton sticks and sheets by an assistant to fill or compress the scleral wound for hemostasis. The compression hemostasis method with cotton sticks and sheets is quite effective on small vessel hemorrhage or scleral surface errhysis. In case of significant

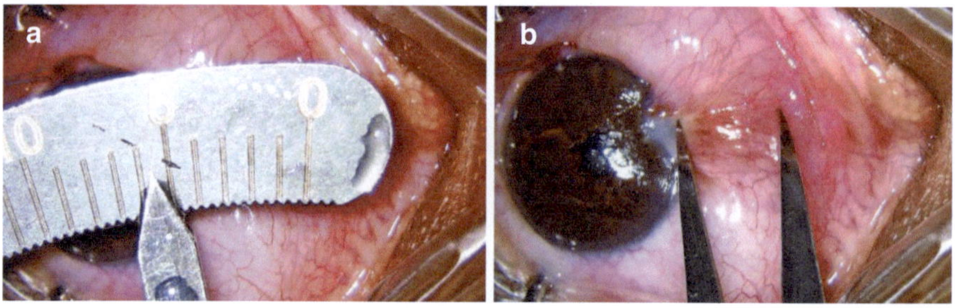

Fig. 6.4 Measurement of excision extension. (**a**) Measure the distance with a gauge; (**b**) the terminus of medial rectus is 5.5 mm from the corneal limbus

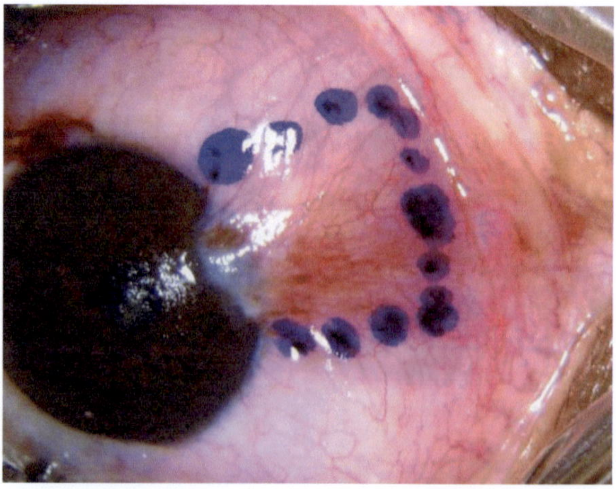

Fig. 6.5 The extent of pterygium excision is labeled using a marker pen, and the length of excision is 5.5 mm from the corneal scleral limbus

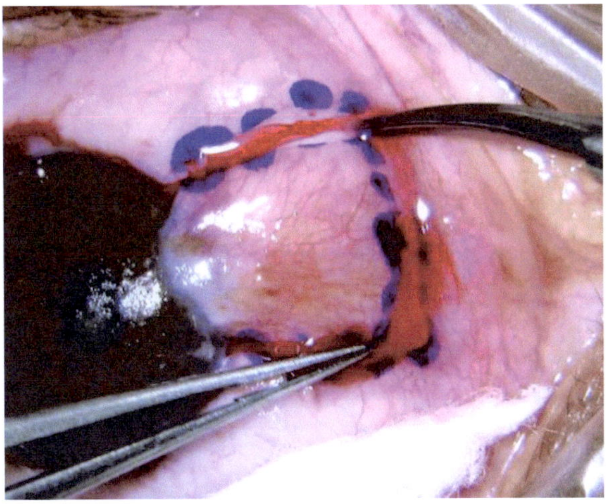

Fig. 6.6 The superficial bulb conjunctiva of pterygium is cut along the labeling line

vascular hemorrhage, large bleeding vessels can be electrocoagulated or cauterized with an bipolar electrocoagulation for hemostasis. If a copper cauterizer is used to cauterize the bleeding vessels for hemostasis, care should be taken that the scleral wound surface cannot be excessively cauterized to avoid scleral avascular necrosis and dissolved perforation. On the premise of no intraoperative injury of medial rectus, the compression hemostasis method with cotton pads is suitable for general bleeding.

Cut the cotton pads soaked with normal saline into a size of 6 mm × 7 mm, place it close to the scleral wound surface for 2–3 min after wringing for hemostasis of scleral errhysis or small vessel hemorrhage (Fig. 6.10).

5. Preparation of superiorly free bulbar conjunctival autograft: Release the eyeball traction wire and instruct the patient to look down (the wire should be guided downward by an assistant if patients cannot cooperate). Beginners can mark the epithelial surface of the upper bulbar conjunctiva with a marker pen, and the skilled operator does not need to measure. Measure according to the gauge or compare the test results with micro-tweezers to make the upper bulbar conjunctival flap, and it is required that no fascia tissue is left or as little as possible under the bulbar conjunctiva (Figs. 6.11 and 6.12).
6. Transplantation and suture of free bulbar conjunctiva autograft: Move the free bulbar conjunctiva graft to the bare sclera with toothless forceps; fix the bulbar conjunctiva on the corneal limbus side on the corneal limbus by contraposition suture, and the bulbar conjunctiva of the fornix part on the bulbar conjunctiva of the lacrimal caruncle region on the graft bed. Suture the four corners of the graft with 10-0 nylon thread for four stitches, which should cover shallow scleral tissue. Fix the transplanted conjunctival graft on the scleral surface with tension, and sew the upper and lower implant beds with the graft bulbar conjunctiva end-to-end continuously or intermittently. Continuous suture or intermittent suture can be performed in the mound of lacrimal area, and a long thread of 5–10 mm

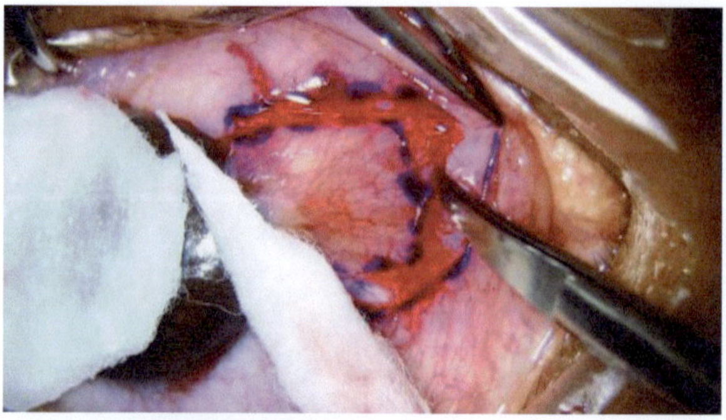

Fig. 6.7 The bulbar conjunctiva is separated from its inferior fascia, at nasal 2 mm, upper and lower 1 mm distance

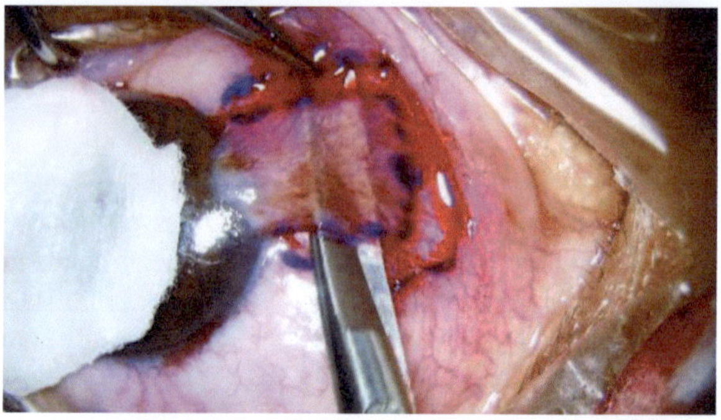

Fig. 6.8 Closed microscissors insert via the upper pterygium under the fascia and separate the pterygium and its inferior sclera along the scleral surface

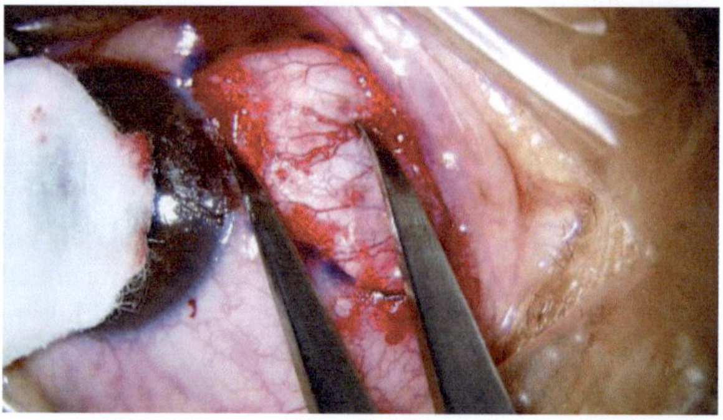

Fig. 6.9 The toothed forceps retains the head part of the pterygium for traction towards the cornea to stretch it, and then excises the pterygium

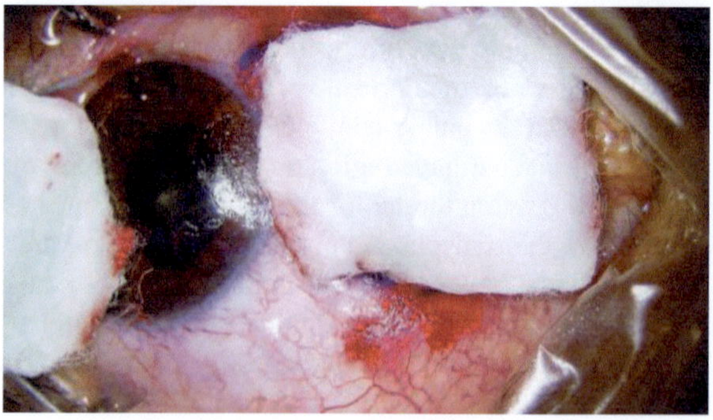

Fig. 6.10 The scleral wound is compressed with the dried saline cotton block, with good hemostatic effect

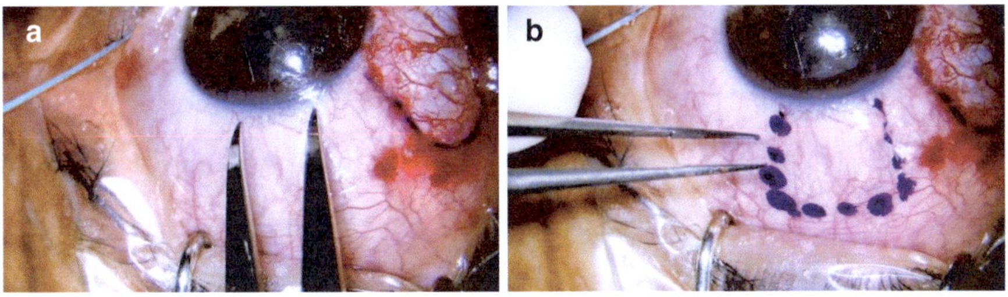

Fig. 6.11 Measurement and marking of sampling range of superior conjunctival flap. (**a**) Measure the width of bulbar conjunctival flap, generally 0.25 mm narrower than the neck of pterygium; (**b**) mark the incision on the epithelial surface of the upper bulbar conjunctiva with a marker

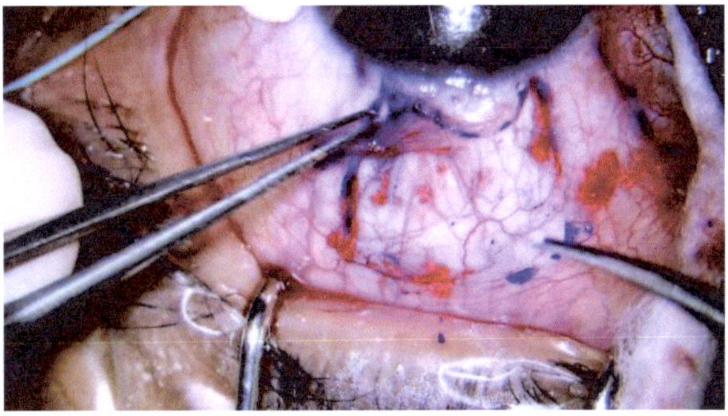

Fig. 6.12 No or little fascial tissue is maintained under the upper bulbar conjunctiva, which is convenient for rapid repair of the upper bulbar conjunctiva without scarring

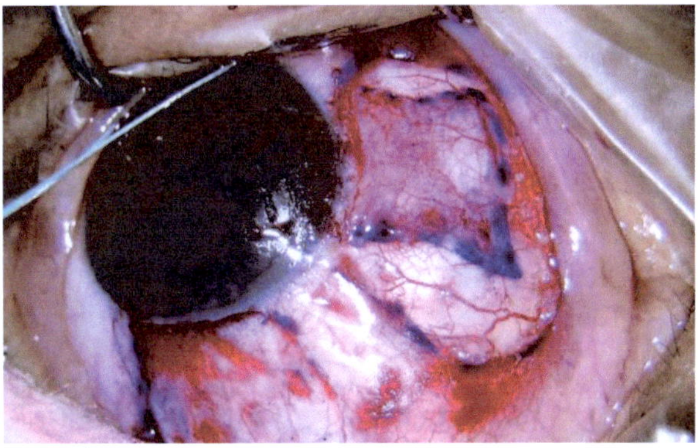

Fig. 6.13 Free and place bulbar conjunctival implant in the contraposition of exposed scleral area

is required to reduce foreign body sensation or stinging caused by the thread (Figs. 6.13, 6.14, and 6.15).

7. Correction of upper bulbar conjunctiva: According to the size of the sample taken from the upper free bulbar conjunctiva, the wound surface of bulbar conjunctiva could be partially sutured or not sutured with 10-0 nylon thread, and bioamnion could be covered when the wound was too large. Because of the upper eyelid coverage, the stem cells of conjunctiva are located in the fornix, and the wound surface is rich in fascia. Generally, the upper bulbar conjunctiva can be repaired within 7–10 days.

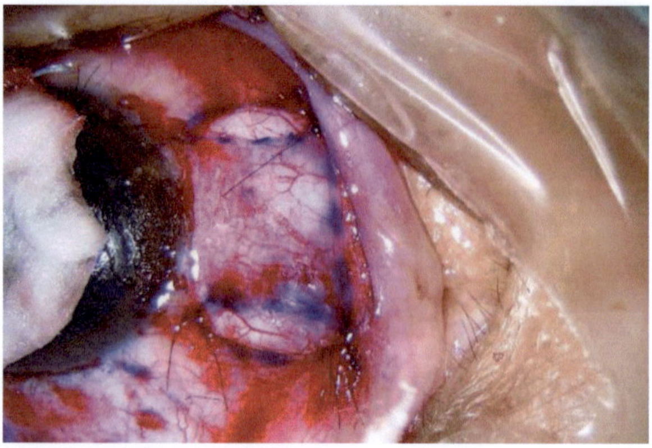

Fig. 6.14 The implant is fixed with the implant bed with superficial scleral tissue at four corners through four sutures, and the implant is fixed on the scleral surface of the operating field

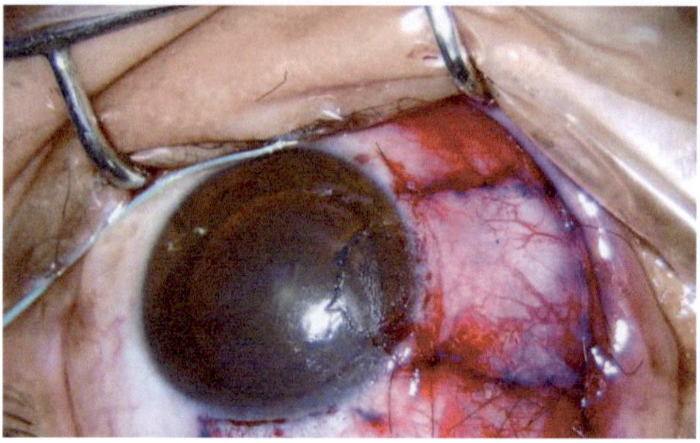

Fig. 6.15 The implant conjunctiva and the implant bed conjunctiva are intermittently or continuously sutured in end-to-end manner, without superficial sclera involved in suturing, and the implant at the corneal limbus may be retreated by 0.2 mm to prevent postoperative implant bulbar conjunctival eminence to form corneal foveas

8. Check: After suturing, it is necessary to check whether the bulbar conjunctiva at the anastomotic site is jointed neatly, whether there is active bleeding under the conjunctiva, and whether the free bulbar conjunctival flap is placed correctly. After the operation is confirmed to be correct, the corneal wound and conjunctival sac are rinsed with normal saline, and the implant is gently squeezed with a medical sponge or a cotton swab to eliminate blood accumulation and fluid accumulation under the conjunctival flap, so that the bulbar conjunctival flap is tightly attached to the sclera.
9. Management of corneal surface wound: Postoperative corneal bare wound will be accompanied by severe pain, and corneal bandage lens can protect the wound and relieve pain. Apply tobramycin and dexamethasone eye cream, bandage for 2–4 h, and then open the operative eyes. Apply the conventional topical application according to the perioperative application (Figs. 6.16 and 6.17).

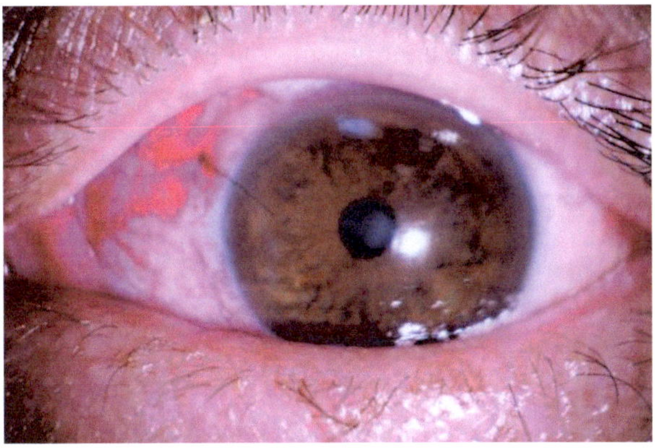

Fig. 6.16 On the second day of postoperative, the corneal bandage lens is placed properly, and the implant is flat through end-to-end anastomosis

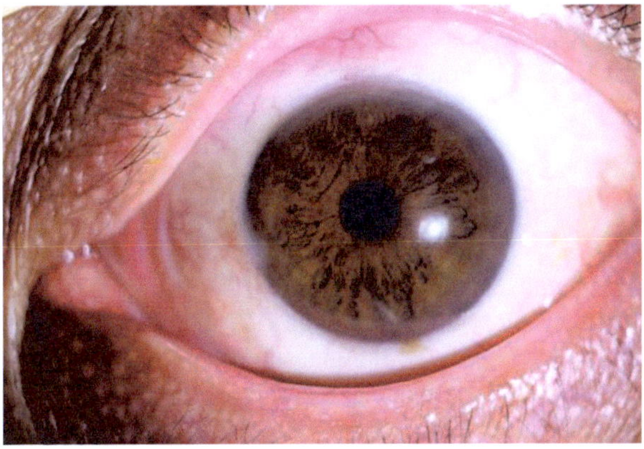

Fig. 6.17 Image of the above-mentioned patient at half and 3 months after general surgery for pterygium, the corneal wound is clean, and the aesthetic grading of the operating field is Grade 2, with good appearance

6.2 Part II: Modified PERFECT for Pterygium

Compared with the conventional pterygium resection with free conjunctival flap autograft mentioned above, this procedure is mainly characterized by a wider excision range. Cornelius et al. treated 60 patients with primary pterygium by pterygium extended removal followed by extended conjunctival transplantation (PERFECT), with a recurrence rate of 1.6% [2]; Hirst et al. treated 1000 patients with primary pterygium using this procedure, in which all tissues except the medial rectus were excised, approximately 14 mm × 14 mm in size, and conjunctival grafts of the corresponding diameter were taken above for sutural closure. Synchronous wire suspending of medial and lateral rectus was required during the operation, and the results showed that the recurrence rate was 0.1%. However, this procedure has not been popularized due to its association with many other complications including strabismus, conjunctival cysts, conjunctival granulomas and corneal ulcers, and due to the long time and strong postoperative discomfort of patients [3].

After several years of improvement, the author fused the advantages of Cornelius to obtain similar surgical results to PERFECT, while eliminating its complications. The surgical resection range of this procedure compared with PERFECT is as follows: upper and lower fascia not exceeding 2 mm outside the conjunctival incision; lacrimal caruncle side not exceeding 3 mm inside the conjunctival incision. There is no intraoperative requirement to free the medial rectus, perturb the muscle, or restrict the ligament, and the surgical wound surface should not exceed 10 mm × 12 mm. Due to the relatively shortened operation time, mild postoperative discomfort for patients, lower postoperative recurrence rate, wider resection range and significant improvement in aesthetic degree, this procedure is known as modified PERFECT. The key steps for improvement include:

1. An extended excision range of pterygium reaching 2.0–3.0 mm after the terminus of medial rectus.
2. No disassociation of medial rectus.
3. Preservation of muscle sheath above the medial rectus.
4. A bulbar conjunctival incision 1.0–1.5 mm anterior to the lacrimal caruncle.

6.2.1 Surgical Indications

This surgical procedure is indicated to primary and recurrent pterygium, especially for giant pterygium with high risk of recurrence, hereditary pterygium in young adults, pterygium with congestion that does not subside after 3 days of hormone use, and mild to moderate recurrent pterygium with no scar or superficial scars. The surgical steps are as follows (Fig. 6.18):

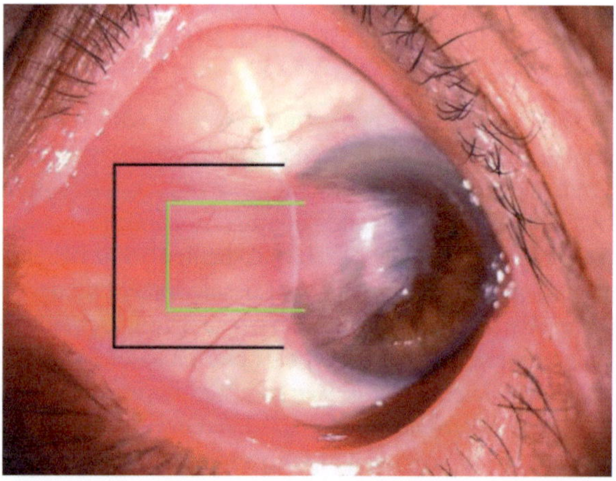

Fig. 6.18 Extent of pterygium excision by general approach and modified PERFECT approach. Green frame refers to the extent of general pterygium excision, and the incision reaches the end of the medial rectus muscle, 5.5 mm away from the corneal limbus. Black frame refers to the extent of modified PERFECT excision approach, the incision reached 1.5 mm in front of the lacrimal caruncle, 7.5 mm away from the corneal limbus

6.2.2 Surgical Steps

1. Anesthesia: See Part I of this chapter for related content (see Figs. 6.1 and 6.2).
2. Fixation of eyeballs: See Part I of this chapter for related content (see Fig. 6.3).
3. Pterygium excision: This procedure focuses on the complete resection of the subconjunctival degenerative fibrous tissue up to (9–10 mm) × (10–12 mm), including the fascia above the rectus muscle, in order to completely eradicate the source of recurrence and obtain a good cosmetic improvement. The excision range of pterygium in modified PERFECT is 2.0–2.5 mm medial to the terminus of medial rectus, 7.0–7.5 mm from the corneal limbus, and the bulbar conjunctival incision 1.5 mm in front of the lacrimal caruncle. This procedure generally requires experience with more than 1000 conventional pterygium surgeries.

   Beginners should first measure the operation distance with a ruler and draw the conjunctival incision line with a marker (experienced people don't need to mark it). Sever the bulbar conjunctiva along the upper and lower margins of pterygium to 1.5 mm in front of the lacrimal caruncle, and disconnect the superficial bulbar conjunctiva above the medial rectus parallel to the corneal limbus. Lift the conjunctiva at the upper, lower, and nasal bulbar conjunctival incisions in sequence, and bluntly exfoliate the inferior and external fascia at 1 mm above and below the incisions and 2 mm within the lacrimal caruncle conjunctiva. Disassociate the bulbar conjunctiva and fascia under the conjunctival incision with closed microscissors and cut it open by about 3 mm with the blades. Care should be taken to protect the sheath of medial rectus. Separation of the bulbar conjunctiva from its underlying fascia ensures extensive removal of the tissue adjacent to the pterygium, which is essential to reduce recurrence and obtain a good appearance.

   After separation of the bulbar conjunctiva and fascia, the pterygium should be separated from the sclera as in conventional pterygium surgery. After separation, the superior and inferior fascia should be cut. Make a scratch on the pterygium head along the corneal surface to the depth of corneal epithelial layer with closed ophthalmic microscissors, clamp the pterygium head with a toothed forceps, and then exfoliate it along the corneal surface to the neck with microscissors. Next, clamp the pterygium head with a toothed forceps again, and bluntly exfoliate the neck of pterygium with closed microscissors until the pterygium is completely dissociated from the corneal surface and limbus, at which time, its three surfaces are completely disassociated and the medial rectus sheath is exposed. It should be noted that severe hemorrhage may be caused by collision of rectus muscle with any instrument.

   Clamp the head of pterygium horizontally with a toothed forceps and pull it towards the cornea for full exposure under a certain tension, and excise the pterygium above the medial rectus with microscissors. The exposed area of the scleral wound depends on the size of pterygium and generally does not exceed (9–10 mm) × (10–12 mm) (Figs. 6.19, 6.20, 6.21, 6.22, and 6.23).
4. Wound hemostasis: See Part I of this chapter for related content (Fig. 6.24).

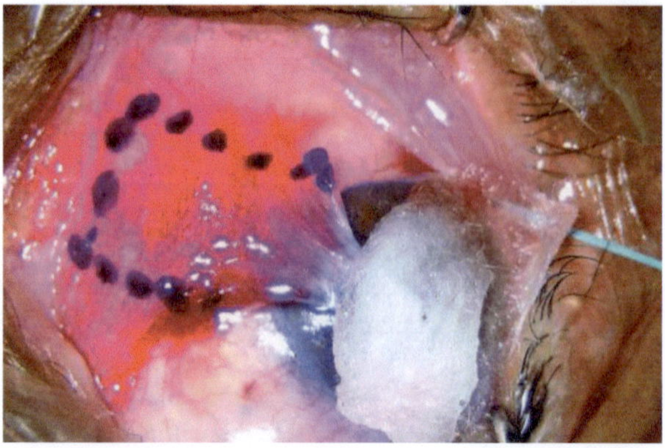

Fig. 6.19 Mark the scope of the bulbar conjunctival incision with a marker, with the nasal side reaching 1.5 mm in front of the lacrimal caruncle

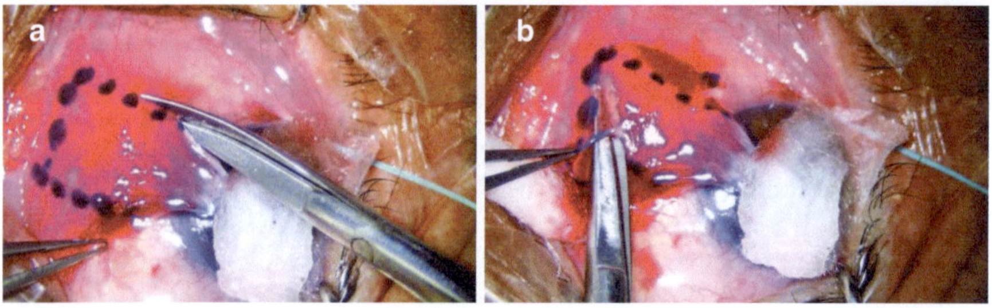

Fig. 6.20 Excision and dissociation of bulbar conjunctiva. (**a**, **b**) Excise the bulbar conjunctiva along the marked line

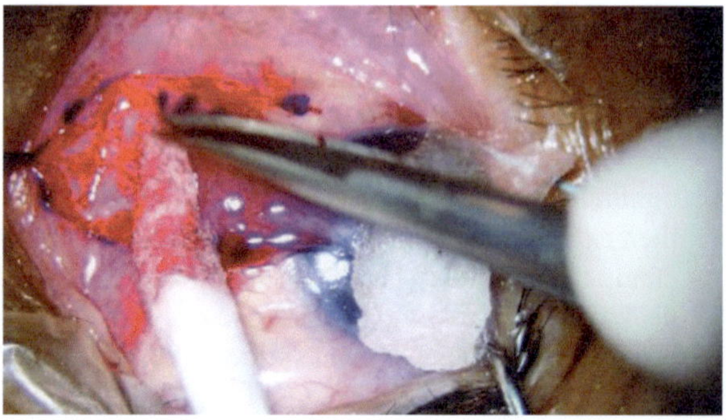

Fig. 6.21 Lifting the bulbar conjunctiva at the incision to separate the conjunctiva from the lower fascia, at upper and lower 1 mm distance and 2 mm inside the conjunctival incision of the lacrimal caruncle

5. Preparation of free bulbar conjunctival autograft: Release the eyeball traction wire and instruct the patient to look down (the wire should be guided downward by an assistant if patients cannot cooperate). Beginners can mark the epithelial surface of the upper bulbar conjunctiva with a marker pen, and the skilled operator does not need to measure. Measure according to the gauge or compare the test results with micro-tweezers to make the upper bulbar conjunctival flap. It is required that no fascia tissue is left or as little as possible under the bulbar con-

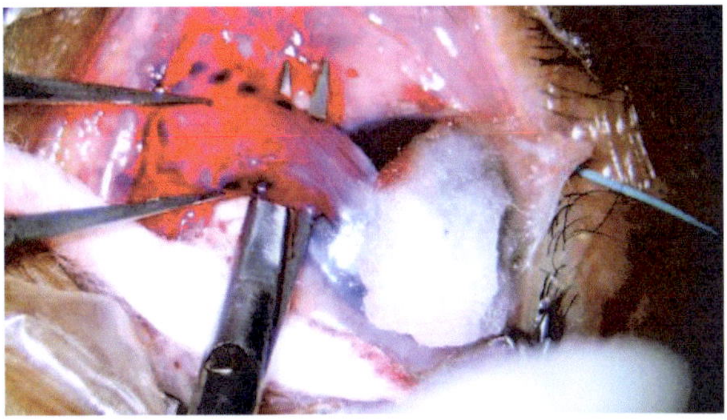

Fig. 6.22 Closed microscissors insert via the upper pterygium under the fascia and separate the pterygium along the scleral surface

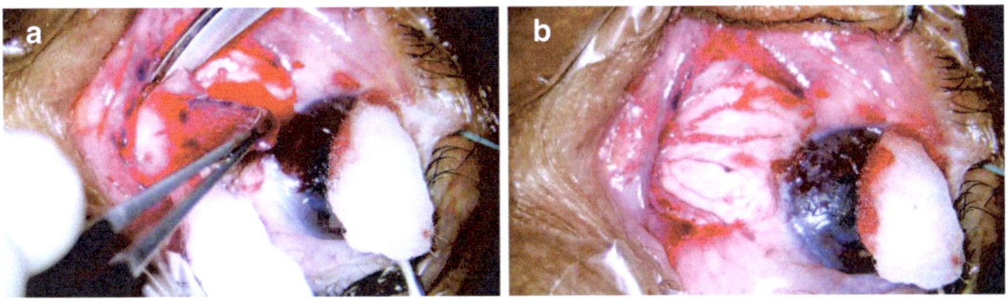

Fig. 6.23 Excision of pterygium. (**a**) Clamp the head of pterygium horizontally with a toothed forceps and pull it towards the cornea for full exposure under a certain tension, and excise the pterygium above the medial rectus with microscissors; (**b**) the scleral surgical area, about (9–10 mm) × (10–12 mm) is exposed after pterygium resection

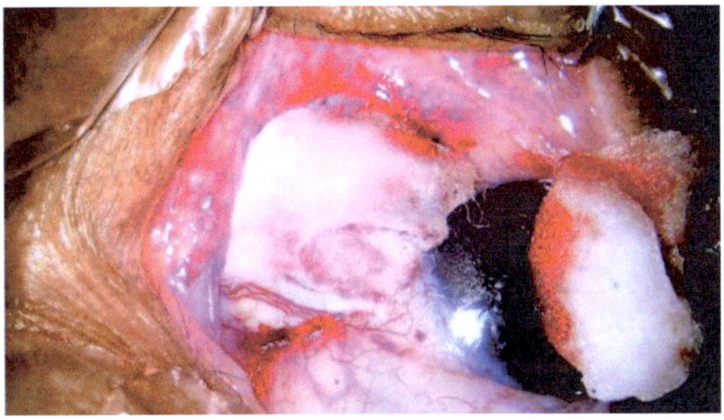

Fig. 6.24 The scleral wound is compressed with the dried saline cotton block for hemostasis

junctiva. The conjunctival flap should be made according to the following principles: 0.25–0.5 mm smaller than the scleral exposed wound, trapezoidal, with no or very little fascia, and close to the limbus but without the need for limbus stem cells (Figs. 6.25 and 6.26).

6. Transplantation and suture of free bulbar conjunctiva autograft: Move the free bulbar conjunctiva graft to the bare sclera with toothless forceps; fix the bulbar conjunctiva on the corneal limbus side on the corneal limbus by contraposition suture, and the bulbar conjunctiva of the fornix part on the bulbar conjunctiva of

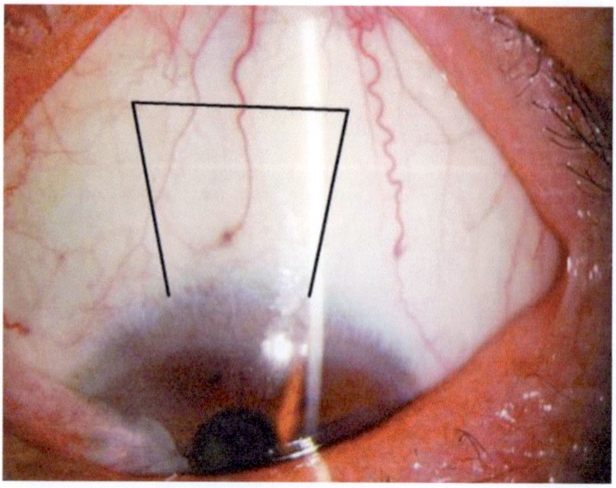

Fig. 6.25 Black line refers to the upper bulbar conjunctival cutting area, the bulbar conjunctival elasticity is good, and the upper bulbar conjunctival flap is smaller than the exposed sclera area

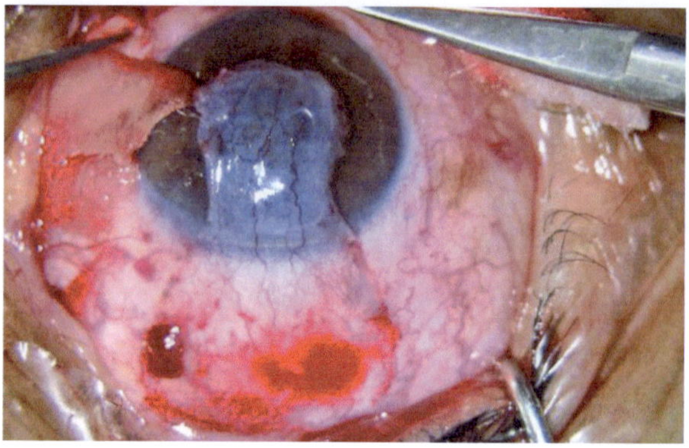

Fig. 6.26 Bulbar conjunctival flap without fascia

the lacrimal caruncle region on the graft bed. Suture the four corners of the graft with 10-0 nylon thread for four stitches, which should cover shallow scleral tissue. The rest of the upper and lower bulbar conjunctiva can be added 1–2 stitches of intermittent suture, or continuous suture. Continuous suture in the lacrimal caruncle area is recommended, and a 5–10 mm long thread should be retained to reduce foreign body sensation or sharp pain.

The graft suture requirements are as follows: (1) The four corners should be firmed sutured with the superficial sclera for four stitches; (2) the graft should be fixed in a tent shape with tension; (3) the graft should be firmly attached and completely cover the scleral wound; (4) the transposed conjunctiva graft should be end-to-end anastomosed with its graft bed; (5) the fascia below the anastomosis should be completely removed; (6) continuous suturing of the conjunctiva on the lacrimal caruncle side can prevent the conjunctival flap at the anastomosis from splitting due to ocular mobility (Figs. 6.27 and 6.28).

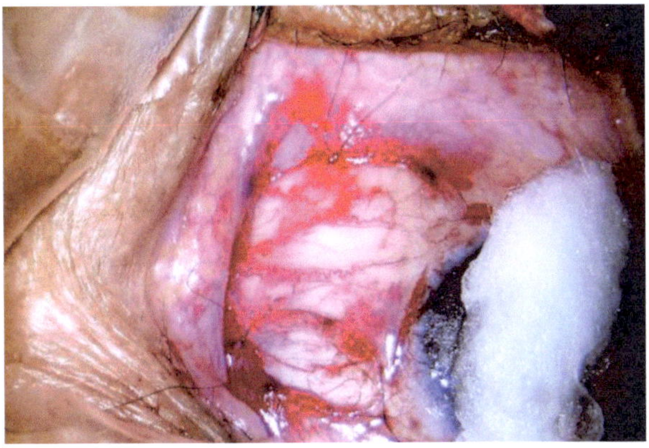

Fig. 6.27 The implant conjunctival limb is aligned with the implant bed conjunctival limbus, implanted intact and fixed with superficial scleral tissue at four corners through four sutures

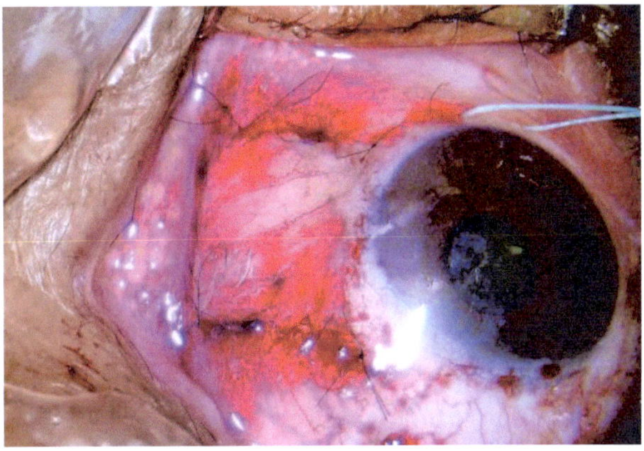

Fig. 6.28 10-0 nylon thread is used to continuously suture the upper, lower and lacrimal caruncle implants and implant bed bulbar conjunctiva

7. Correction of upper bulbar conjunctiva: According to the size of the sample taken from the upper free bulbar conjunctiva, the wound surface of bulbar conjunctiva could be partially sutured or not sutured with 10-0 nylon thread, and bioamnion could be covered when the wound was too large. Because of the upper eyelid coverage, the stem cells of conjunctiva are located in the fornix, and the wound surface is rich in fascia. Generally, the upper bulbar conjunctiva can be repaired within 7–10 days if corneal and conjunctival epithelial healing can be accelerated by covering bioamnion (see Part III).
8. Check: After suturing, it is necessary to flush the operation area with normal saline and check whether there is hematoma in the lacrimal caruncle area.
9. Management of corneal surface wound: Postoperative corneal bare wound will be accompanied by severe pain. To relieve the pain, we will apply corneal bandage lens, tobramycin and dexamethasone eye cream, and bandage for 2–4 h; then open the operative eyes to apply the conventional topical application, according to the perioperative application (Figs. 6.29, 6.30, 6.31, 6.32, and 6.33).

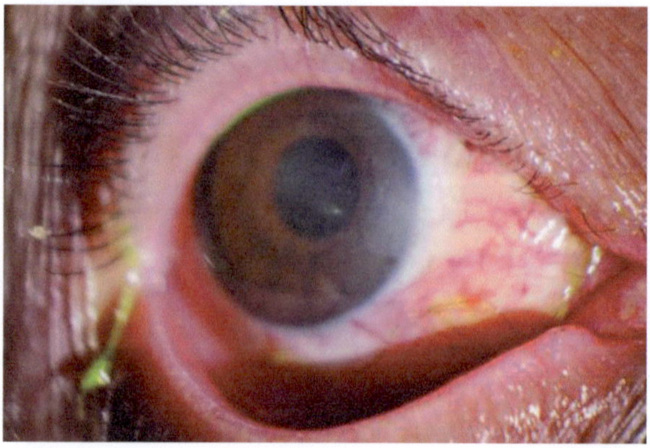

Fig. 6.29 Image of the patient on the seventh day after modified PERFECT surgery, conjunctival flap is flat, sutures are placed properly, corneal epithelium is repaired

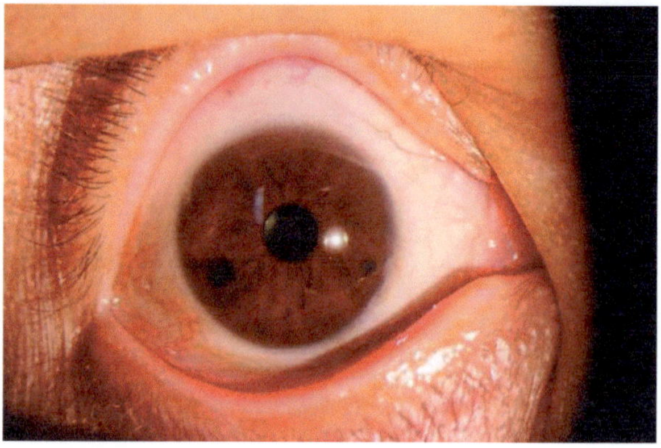

Fig. 6.30 Appearance of the same patient at 6 months after modified PERFECT surgery, aesthetic grading is Grade 1, with normal appearance

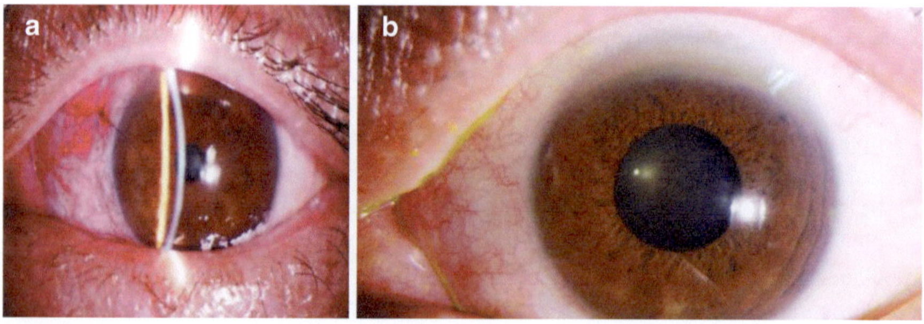

Fig. 6.31 Postoperative photo of modified PERFECT. (**a**) The picture taken on the next day after modified PERFECT surgery showed that the bandage lens was in place, and the patient had no wound pain; (**b**) 3 months after modified PERFECT operation in the same patient

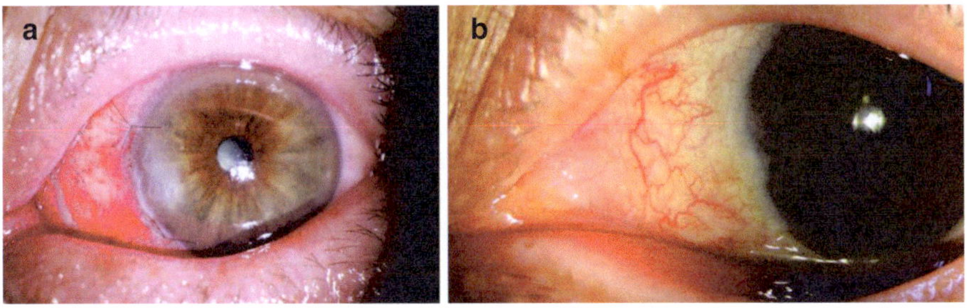

Fig. 6.32 Postoperative photo of modified PERFECT. (**a**) The picture taken on the next day after modified PERFECT surgery showed that the bandage lens was in place, and the patient had no wound pain; (**b**) 3 months after modified PERFECT operation in the same patient

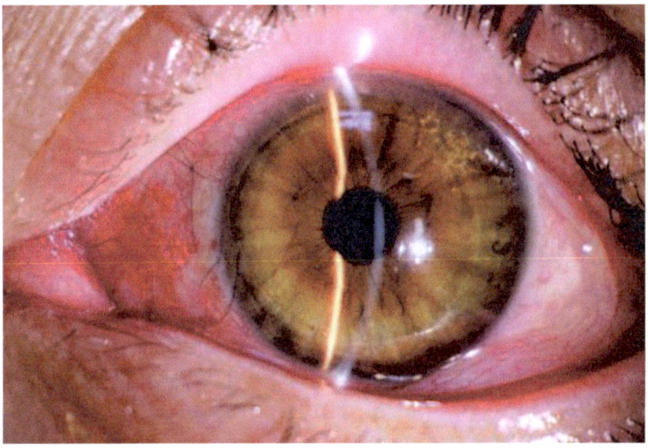

Fig. 6.33 The picture taken on the next day after modified PERFECT surgery showed that the bandage lens was in place, and the patient had no wound pain

6.3 Part III: Modified PERFECT for Pterygium with Bioamnion Covering

The management of corneal wounds after pterygium surgery is often ignored by some surgeons. However, wound pain not only brings unacceptable pain to patients, but also leads to corneal infection, delayed epithelial healing, and prolonged inflammation due to wound exposure, which may eventually accelerate the recurrence of pterygium and related complications after surgery. The management of corneal wounds after pterygium surgery needs to be highly valued by clinicians.

There are two ways to manage corneal wounds after pterygium surgery: (1) Covering the corneal wound with a corneal bandage lens to protect the wound and relieve pain; (2) using a 10 mm × 15 mm bioamnion to cover the corneal wound, which can not only relieve wound pain, accelerate corneal epithelial repair and inhibit scar formation, but also reduce inflammatory response, making the postoperative appearance of pterygium more beautiful and the recurrence rate lower.

Modified PERFECT with bandage lens covering is widely known as "pterygium bigeminy", i.e., extensive excision of pterygium with free conjunctival flap autograft. The pterygium surgery with bioamnion covering following modified PERFECT is called "pterygium trilogy", i.e., extensive pterygium resection + free conjunctival flap autograft + bioamnion covering. This part focuses on the trilogy of pterygium.

6.3.1 Bioamnion Functions

Bioamnion covers corneal wound: Bioamnion is the innermost semitransparent membrane of fetal membranes, which does not contain blood vessels, lymphatic vessels and nerve fibers, and is full of toughness and has therapeutic functions that cannot be achieved by multiple drugs. Bioamnion is a finished amnion made from multiple layers of fresh amnion through special physical processing, which is sterilized by irradiation with cobalt 60 and retains all the functions of fresh amnion. Bioamnion can be stored at room temperature, and it is convenient to transport. It has been commercialized and mass-produced, which has relieved the troubles and many risks of self-made amnion for ophthalmology clinic. Bioamnion can be used in clinical ophthalmology for glaucoma filtering bleb repair, conjunctival sac shaping for eye reshaping, etc. It is more widely used in ocular surface diseases, especially in pterygium surgery. Bioamnion has the following functions:

1. Alleviate inflammatory reaction and accelerate inflammation regression after pterygium operation: Bioamnion contains various protease inhibitors, such as trypsin, fibrin, cathepsin, collagenase, etc., so as to reduce inflammatory reaction. The authors compared the patients whose corneal wounds were covered with or without bioamnion after modified PERFECT surgery. The patients whose corneal wounds were covered with bioamnion had faster envy regression time, faster corneal epithelial repair and smoother conjunctival wound after surgery (Figs. 6.34 and 6.35).
2. Relieve wound pain: Large epithelial defects in corneal wounds after pterygium surgery can cause severe pain in corneal wounds. There have been reports of addiction after analgesic use of pethidine due to postoperative wound pain in pterygium (addiction per se or addiction to postoperative analgesia, for the record). Nevertheless, the corneal wound after pterygium surgery must be properly treated, because pain not only increases the pain of patients, but also may lead to wound infection, delayed healing of corneal epithelium, etc.
3. Inhibition of angiogenesis and reduction of scar formation: The amniotic basement layer can inhibit the proliferation of transforming growth factor signals, inhibit the proliferation and differentiation of fibroblasts, inhibit the proliferation of new blood vessels, and reduce scar formation. The postoperative anastomosis of pterygium usually leads to poor appearance due to fibrous hyperplasia and scar formation. For the same surgical procedure, the cases combined with bioamniotic covering have a more pleasing appearance (Figs. 6.36 and 6.37).

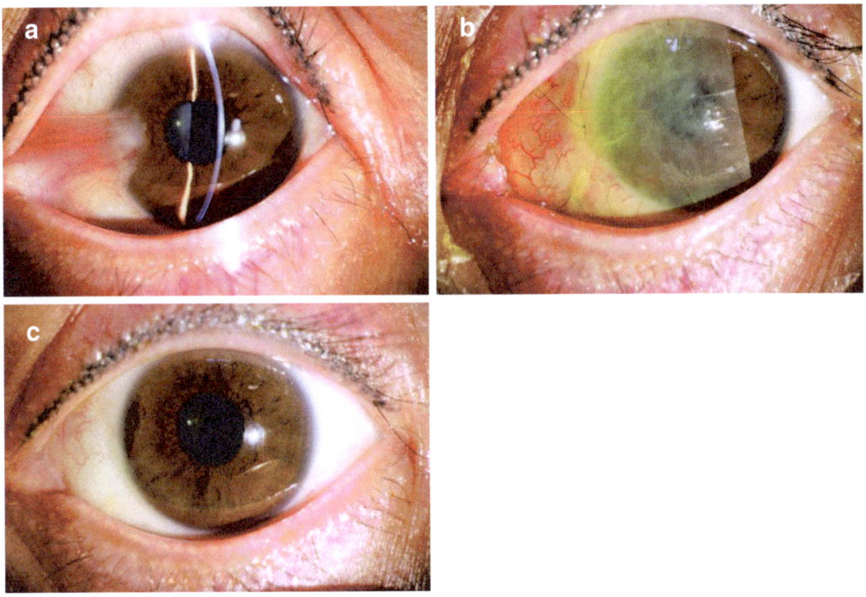

Fig. 6.34 External eye image before and after modified PERFECT combined with biological amniotic membrane covering (triple surgery). (**a**) Before surgery, primary pterygium congestion is relived after 3-day anti-inflammatory therapy; (**b**) 7 days after triple surgery, biological amniotic membrane is placed properly; (**c**) appearance of the patient at 3 weeks after triple surgery

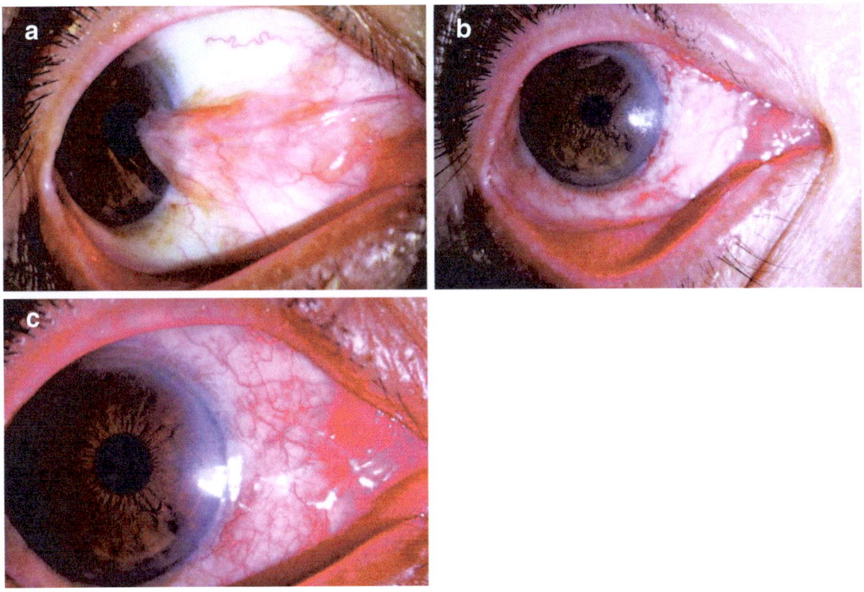

Fig. 6.35 External eye image before and after modified PERFECT (double surgery). (**a**) Before surgery, primary pterygium is at quiescent phase; (**b**) on the second day after double surgery, bandage lends are placed properly; (**c**) appearance of the patient at 1 month after double surgery

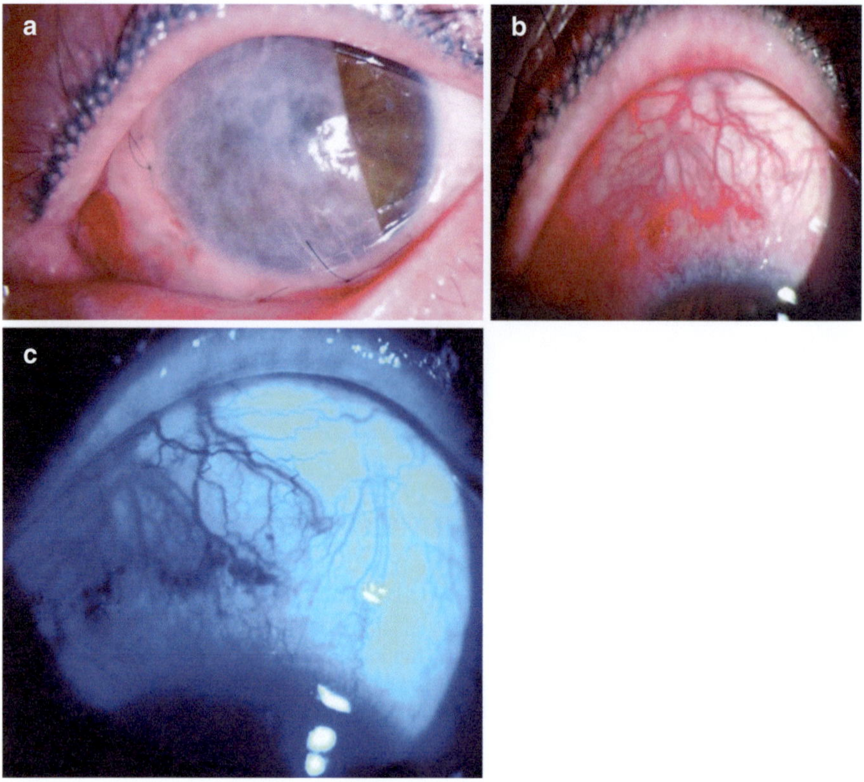

Fig. 6.36 Postoperative wound healing of modified PERFECT with bioamnion covering (trilogy). (**a**) Bioamnion was used for postoperative cover; (**b**) on POD7, after the bioamnion was removed by suture removal, the complete repair of the upper bulbar conjunctiva, and smooth wound surface free of scars were observed. (**c**) No epithelial defect on fluorescein staining was noted

4. Acceleration of corneal epithelial repair and inhibition of fibrogenesis: The amniotic basement layer contains a large number of different collagen fibers, mainly types I, III, IV, V and VII, which can be used as a bridge scaffold for tissue repair. The amniotic basement membrane used for covering corneal wound can strengthen the adhesion of epithelial cells, promote the proliferation and differentiation of epithelial cells and prevent the apoptosis of epithelial cells, thus being beneficial to ocular surface reconstruction after pterygium surgery.
5. Antiviral and antibacterial effects: Human defensins produced by bioamnion, which are widely expressed on the mucosal surface, are the main components of vertebrate natural antibacterial substances; bioamnion tissue graft can synthesize and secrete six complement proteins to participate in local defense reactions, so human bioamnion has mild non-specific antiviral and antibacterial effects.
6. Multiple growth factors: Bioamnion contains multiple growth factors that promote the differentiation, transformation, proliferation and migration of stem cells, as well as the recovery of limbal stem cells after pterygium surgery.

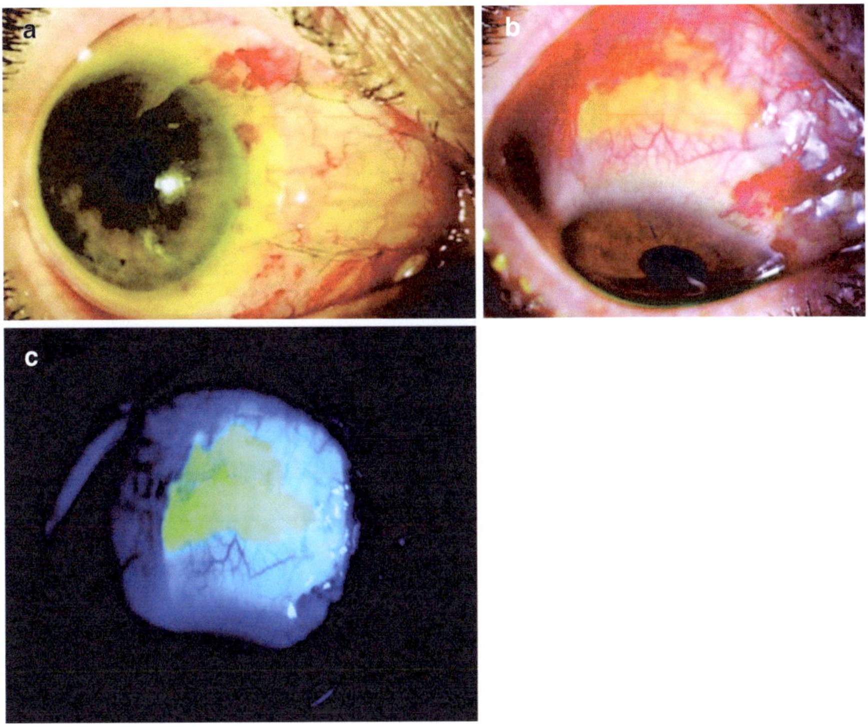

Fig. 6.37 Postoperative wound healing of modified PERFECT (bigeminy). (**a**) Covered with bandage lenses after surgery; (**b**) on POD7, the upper bulbar conjunctiva was not completely healed, and superficial scar formation of conjunctiva could be seen; (**c**) fluorescein staining was positive

7. Non-rejection of allogeneic bioamnion: Bioamnion has extremely low antigenicity because it does not express HLAA, B and DR, and hardly induces rejection.

6.3.2 Indications

1. Moderate, severe and giant pterygium (grade 2–4) with >3 mm invasion of the corneal limbus.
2. Pterygium in patients particularly sensitive to pain.
3. Same as the indications for modified perfect pterygium excision.

The following two precautions should be indicated to patients before surgery:

1. After surgery, the cornea in the pupil area will have a temporary vision loss due to bioamnion covering, lasting about 5–7 days; the bioamnion will dissolve spontaneously after the wound corneal epithelium is repaired. In a few cases, the bioamnion has not dissolved and fallen off within 7–10 days and the corneal

wound epithelium has been repaired, the bioamnion should be removed together with the suture removal.

2. The suture used for fixation of bioamnion may cause mild foreign body sensation, so patients should be instructed to blink frequently to make the suture more fit to the eyes, so as to reduce discomfort. If necessary, bandage lenses can be added to the bioamnion to prolong the stay time of the bioamnion on the corneal surface and improve the comfort.

6.3.3 *Surgical Steps*

Steps 1–8 of this procedure are the same as those of the modified PERFECT (extensive pterygium excision with free conjunctival flap autograft) in the Part II of this chapter. The surgical steps of bioamnion covering are as follows:

1. Size of bioamnion: Select one bioamnion with the size of 10 mm × 15 mm.
2. Covering time: After extensive excision of pterygium with free conjunctival flap autograft, bioamnion is covered on the wounds of cornea and superior bulbar conjunctiva.
3. Coverage: Completely cover the corneal wound, and cover about 1/3 of the area of conjunctiva wound.
4. Fixation method: Suture the bioamnion with 10-0 nylon thread for four stitches to fix it on the scleral side of the upper and lower cornea and scleral margin, which should ensure that the bioamnion tightly wraps the corneal wound (Figs. 6.38, 6.39, 6.40, 6.41, 6.42, 6.43, 6.44, 6.45, and 6.46).
5. Coverage with bandage lenses: corneal bandage lens can be covered on bioamnion after the bioamnion suture is completed.

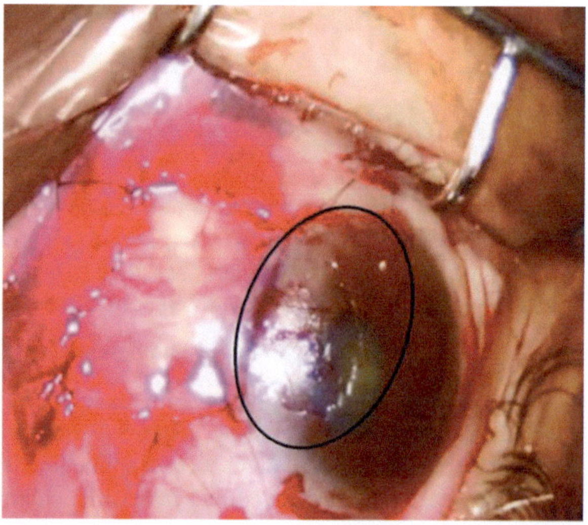

Fig. 6.38 Corneal wounds exposed after the completion of wide excision of pterygium combined with autologous free conjunctival flap transplantation (within black oval circle)

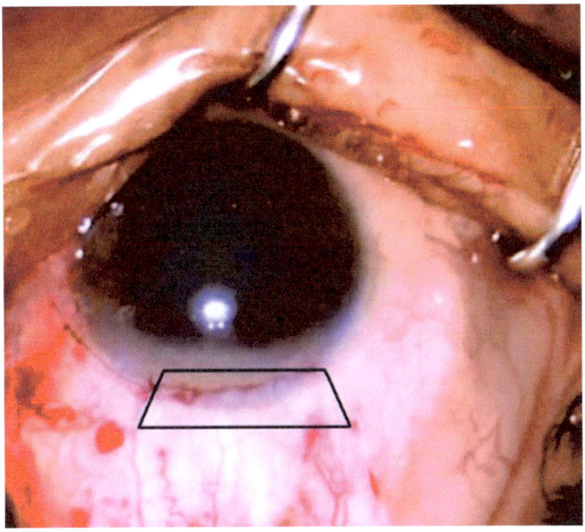

Fig. 6.39 Upper corneal wounds exposed after the completion of wide excision of pterygium combined with autologous free conjunctival flap transplantation, amniotic covering 1/3 of the area (black line range)

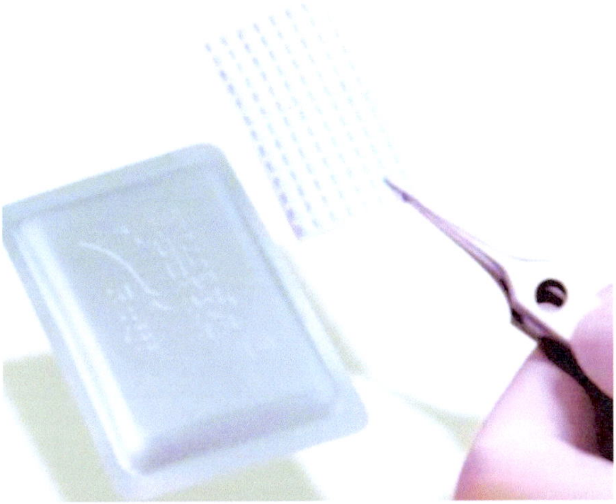

Fig. 6.40 Biological amniotic membrane, convex surface is the basal surface, convex side facing down and adhering to the corneal wound

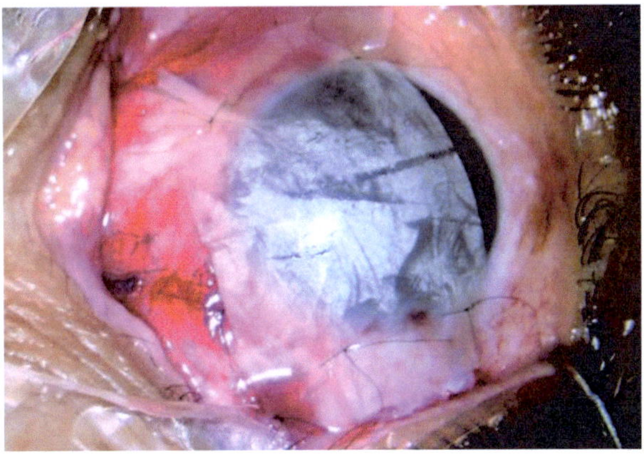

Fig. 6.41 Screenshot of the surgical video, biological amniotic membrane covers and wraps the corneal wound, and the upper conjunctival wound covers 1/3 of the area

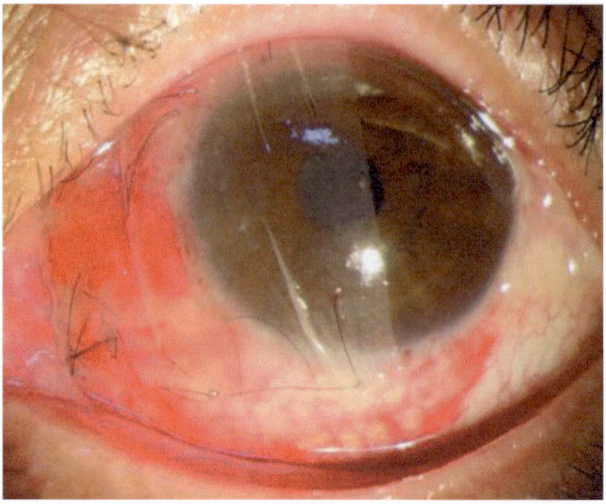

Fig. 6.42 Protomerite image on postoperative 2 days, biological amniotic membrane covers and wraps the corneal wound, and the upper conjunctival wound covers 1/3 of the area

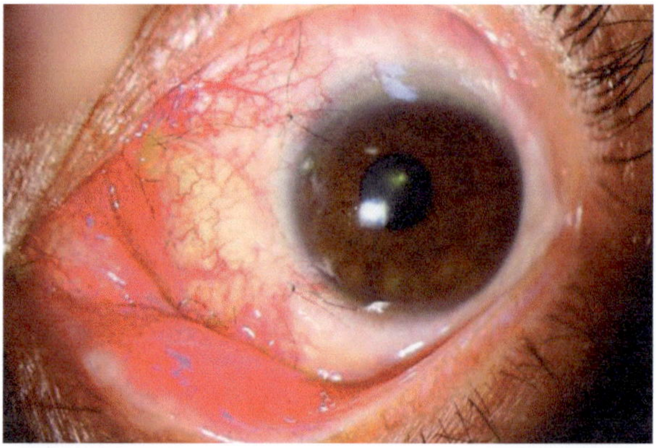

Fig. 6.43 Biological amniotic membrane is dissolved when the patient goes to the hospital for suture removal on the seventh day after triple surgery. The corneal wound is repaired and fluorescein staining is negative

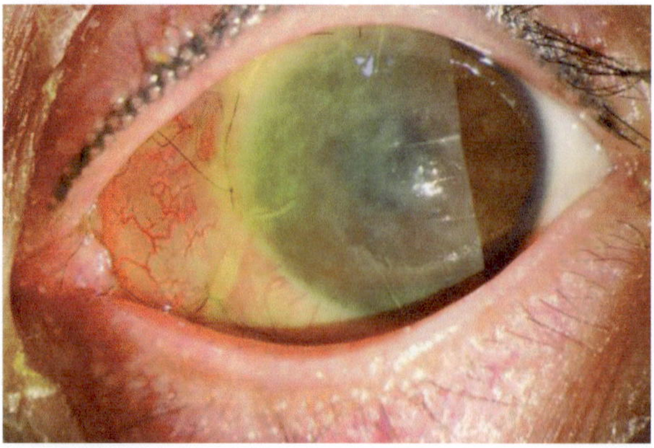

Fig. 6.44 Biological amniotic membrane is placed properly when the patient goes to the hospital for suture removal on the seventh day after triple surgery. After removing the biological amniotic membrane, corneal and conjunctival wound epithelium is repaired, and fluorescein staining is negative

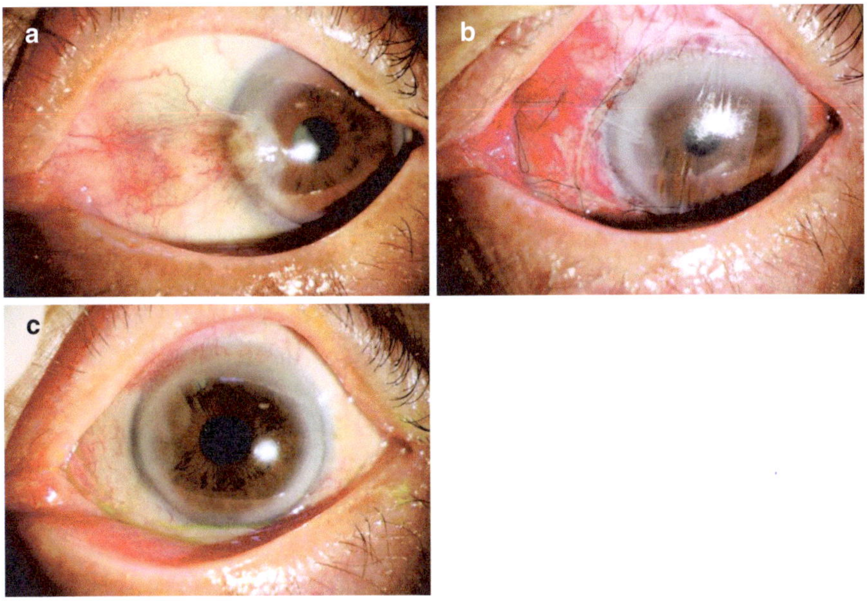

Fig. 6.45 External eye image before and after modified PERFECT combined with biological amniotic membrane covering (triple surgery). (**a**) Preoperative (quiescent phase) of primary pterygium; (**b**) images on the first day of postoperative; (**c**) postoperative 6 months

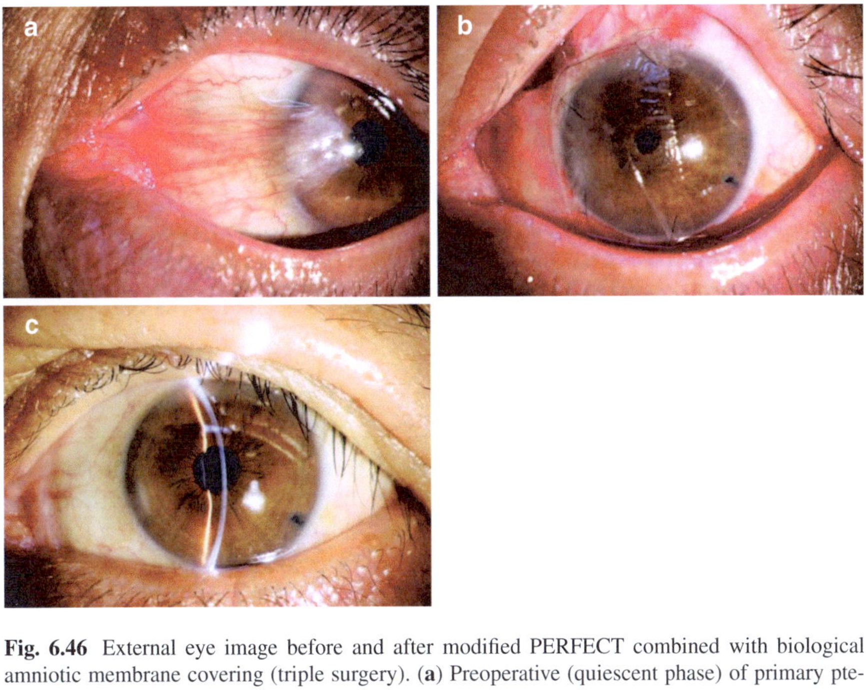

Fig. 6.46 External eye image before and after modified PERFECT combined with biological amniotic membrane covering (triple surgery). (**a**) Preoperative (quiescent phase) of primary pterygium; (**b**) images on the first day of postoperative; (**c**) images at postoperative 1.5 years

6.4 Part IV: Conventional Pterygium Excision with Bioamnion Graft

After years of clinical observation, pterygium excision with bioamnion transplantation has been proved to have the advantages of low recurrence rate, quick wound repair and slight postoperative reaction. However, for pterygium in grade 3 or 4, with a particularly hypertrophic body, or with a familial hereditary predisposition, modified PERFECT is generally necessary. Due to a large exposed area of the sclera, bioamnion transplantation alone (especially single-layer fresh bioamnion) cannot guarantee that the epithelium of the scleral wound in the operation area will be completely repaired before amnion dissolution, so this operation has certain limitation.

6.4.1 Indications

1. Same as those for conventional pterygium excision with free conjunctival flap autograft.
2. Pterygium requiring or following glaucoma filtration surgery.
3. Cases of double-headed or recurrent pterygium secondary to giant pterygium with insufficient conjunctival autografts.

6.4.2 Surgical Points and Steps

After conventional pterygium resection, bioamnion is used instead of free conjunctival flap graft in the scleral surgery area, which does not disturb the adjacent conjunctiva and maintains ocular surface homeostasis. The scleral wound covered with bioamnion transplantation should not be of excessive area, and pterygium resection should cover the range of 0.5 mm in front of the rectus muscle and 5.0 mm from the corneal limbus to ensure that the scleral wound epithelium has been repaired during aminolysis.

The specific steps are as follows:

For Steps 1–4, see the related content of conventional pterygium surgery in Part I of this chapter.

5. Preparation of bioamnion autograft: Based on the size of scleral bare surface, tailor the bioamnion to an autograft 1.0–1.5 mm bigger than the scleral wound, measure with a gauge or mark along that scleral wound surface with a sterilized marker, then cover the scleral wound with bioamnion and slightly compress it. The indentation left on the bibioamnion is the size of the scleral wound. Cut at 1.0–1.5 mm outside the indentation, and the graft should be placed under the conjunctiva of the graft bed during bioamnion transplantation (Figs. 6.47, 6.48, and 6.49).

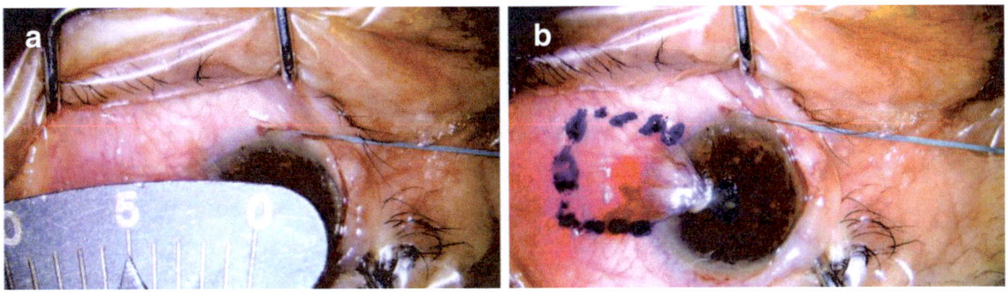

Fig. 6.47 Incision size of common pterygium excision with bioamnion graft. (**a**) Measure the incision length with a gauge (the incision is located 0.5 mm in front of the terminus of medial rectus and 5 mm away from the corneal limbus); (**b**) select the primary pterygium of grade 1 and 2

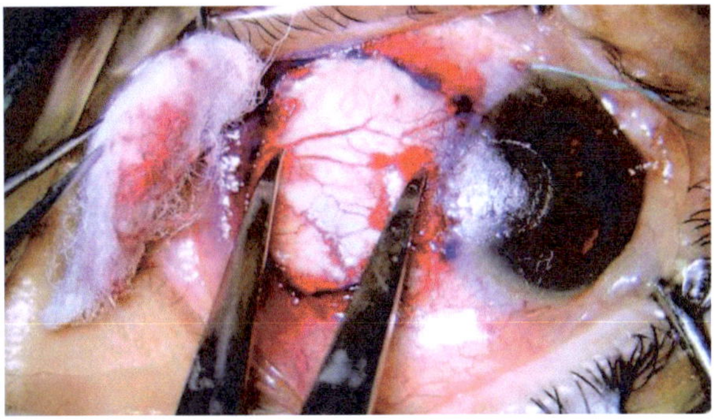

Fig. 6.48 5 mm distance from corneal limbus to the front of rectus terminus

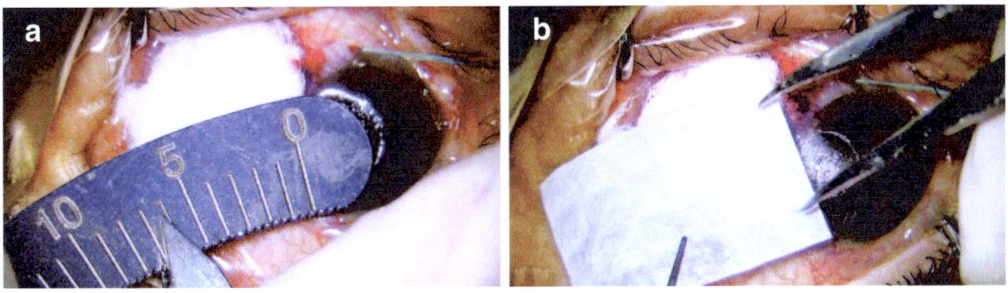

Fig. 6.49 Bioamnion 1.5 mm larger than the incision. (**a**) The tailored bioamnion is 1.5 mm larger than scleral wound; (**b**) measure the size of bioamnion, 1.5 mm larger than the surgical area

6. Transplantation and suture of bioamnion autograft: Clamp the tailored bioamnion graft with a tooted microforceps and move it to the exposed sclera; after wetting with normal saline, insert the bioamnion with its convex facing downward into the graft bed and 1.0–11.5 mm below the conjunctival incision.

   Tightly attach to the sclera, cover the implantation bulbar conjunctiva over the bioamnion and tidy the implantation bulbar conjunctiva. Interruptedly suture the corneal limbus and the four corners in front of the terminus of rectus muscle with 10-0 nylon thread for four stitches in total, which should be sutured along with the superficial sclera and in sequence of amnion (entry)—sclera—amnion—

conjunctiva (exit). In addition to these 4 stitches, interruptedly suture the rest of upper and lower parts in the same way for 1–2 stitches. Either mattress suture for two stitches or interrupted suture is performed on the lacrimal caruncle. A 5–10 mm long thread should be retained to reduce the foreign body sensation or tingling (Figs. 6.50, 6.51, 6.52, and 6.53).

7. Check: After suturing, check for smoothness of the bioamnion, firmness of sutures, pressure on the bioamnion imposed by bulbar conjunctiva, active bleeding under the bioamnion in the surgical area, damage to the bioamnion,

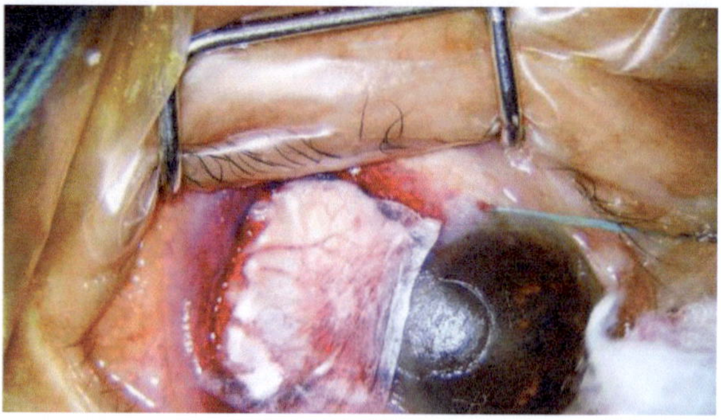

Fig. 6.50 Biological amniotic membrane convex side is facing down, moistened using normal saline

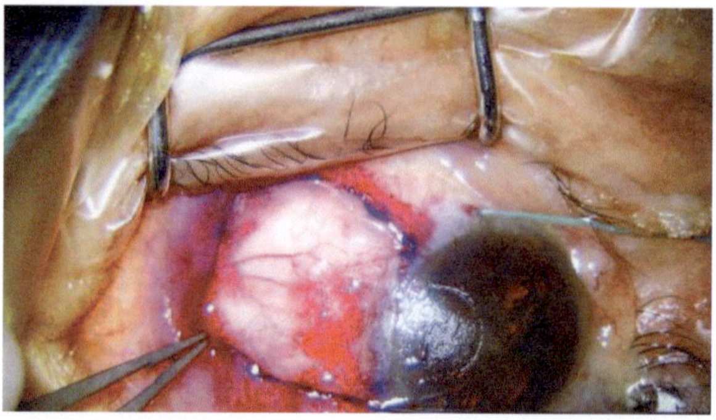

Fig. 6.51 The amniotic membrane is inserted into the conjunctival incision, and the bulbar conjunctiva covers the amniotic membrane

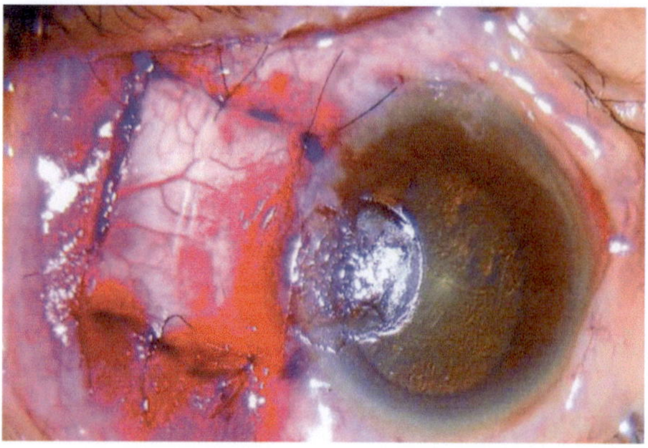

Fig. 6.52 Three intermittent sutures for upper and lower incisions, two mattress sutures for nasal side

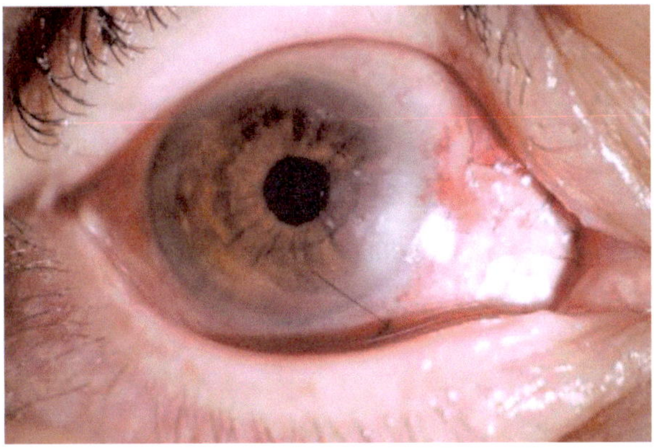

Fig. 6.53 After the surgery completes, corneal wound covers bandage lens to relieve postoperative wound pain

and firm adhesion to the sclera. Rinse the wound surface with normal saline, and squeeze any blood or effusion under the bioamnion on the sclera surface by gently pressing with an absorbent sponge, so that it can better adhere to the scleral wound surface.

8. Management of corneal wound surface: Wear corneal bandage lenses to protect the postoperative bare wound and relieve pain (See Fig. 6.53).

6.5 Part V: Extensive Pterygium Excision with Superficial Conjunctival Flap Transposition

Some scholars once believed that pterygium was actually the proliferation of degenerative fibrous tissue under the conjunctival epithelial layer, without affecting the involved conjunctiva and epithelium. Conventional excision of pterygium usually involves the bulbar conjunctiva on the surface of pterygium body. Many excised bulbar conjunctivae have excellent color, elasticity and luster, and can they be reused? Jap et al. [4] performed a modified conjunctival flap transplantation in a group of patients who cannot be sampled for the superior conjunctival flap by conventional approaches, in which the conjunctival flap from the pterygium surface was transposed by 180° for covering the scleral exposed area (conjunctival rotation autograft, CRA) and a low recurrence rate after excision of pterygium was observed.

Since 2016, the author has performed CRA on more than 50 patients with primary pterygium who could not be sampled for bulbar conjunctiva from the upper and lower parts of pterygium. No postoperative recurrence was observed temporarily, but the patients suffered from long-term mild conjunctival congestion in the surgical area.

6.5.1 Indications

1. Patients with pterygium who have undergone filtration surgery for glaucoma.
2. Patients with both nasal and temporal pterygium.
3. Patients with pterygium who have no access to the superior bulbar conjunctival flap.
4. Elderly patients with pterygium.

6.5.2 Surgical Steps

1. Anesthesia: See Part I of this chapter for related content (see Figs. 6.1 and 6.2).
2. Fixation of eyeballs: See Part I of this chapter for related content (see Fig. 6.3).
3. Preparation of superficial bulbar conjunctival flap at the pterygium corpus: Mark the incision position on the superficial conjunctiva with a marker, and sever the superficial bulbar conjunctiva at the lower, upper, nasal and temporal sides successively along the labeled line at the corneal limbus to 1.5 mm in front of the lacrimal caruncle with microscissors. Penetrate the microscissors into the superficial conjunctiva from the upper conjunctiva incision to separate the superficial bulbar conjunctiva from its lower fascia and dissociate the bulbar conjunctiva on the lacrimal caruncle side; then mark the two corners of the superficial conjunctival flap on the lacrimal caruncle side with 10-0 nylon suture, and mark the center of the epithelial surface of the superficial conjunctiva flap with a marker.

   Hold the labeled line with toothed forceps and lift the superficial conjunctival flap. While separating the subflap fascia, peel the superficial conjunctival flap away from the corneal limbus towards the corresponding direction. Cut the bulbar conjunctiva on the surface layer of pterygium along the marking line, so that the bulbar conjunctiva flap on the surface layer of pterygium is completely free. Lay it flat on the wet saline gauze, clean the residual fascia on the surface of the bulbar conjunctiva flap, fold the saline gauze, cover the implant, and place it in a sterile bowl for use (Figs. 6.54, 6.55, 6.56, 6.57, 6.58, 6.59, and 6.60).

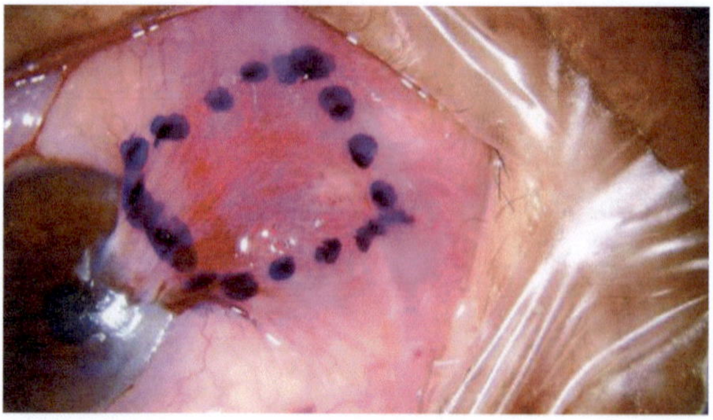

Fig. 6.54 The extent of superficial conjunctival excision of the mattress is labeled using a marker pen

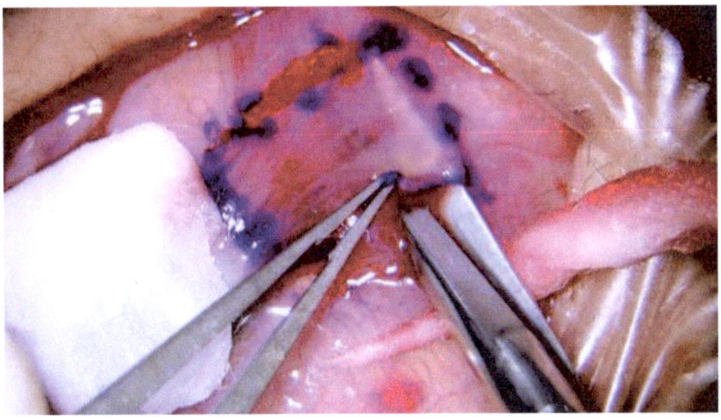

Fig. 6.55 The superficial bulbar conjunctiva is cut and separated from its inferior fascia at nasal 1.5 mm from the lacrimal caruncle

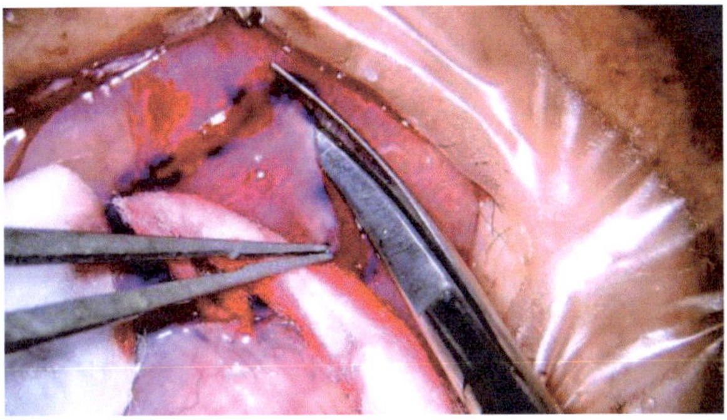

Fig. 6.56 The superficial bulb conjunctiva of pterygium is cut in front of the lacrimal caruncle

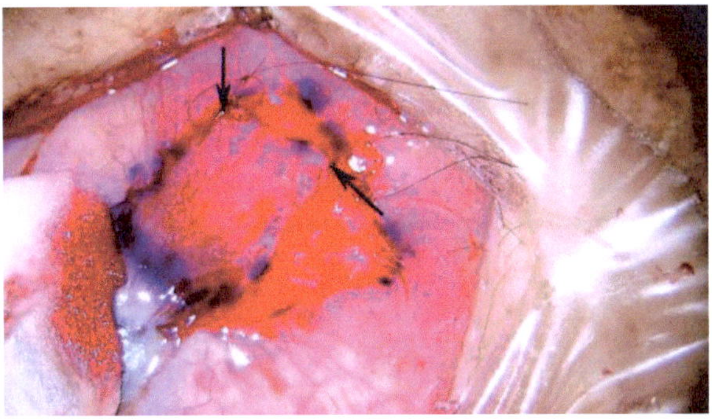

Fig. 6.57 Two corners of the superficial conjunctiva of the pterygium at lacrimal caruncle side is marked with 10-0 nylon thread (black arrow)

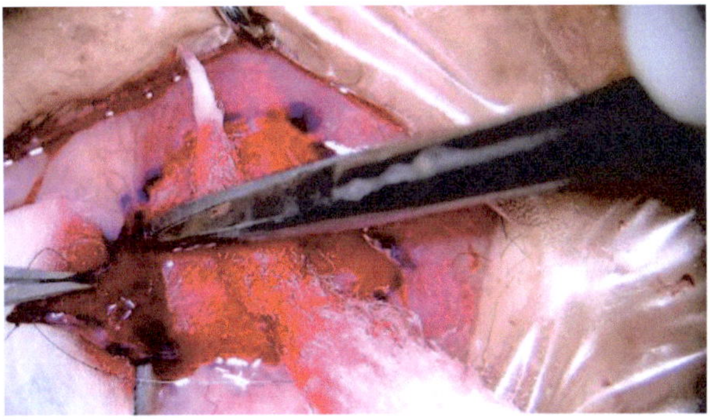

Fig. 6.58 Patiently separate the superficial conjunctival flap towards the neck part of the pterygium

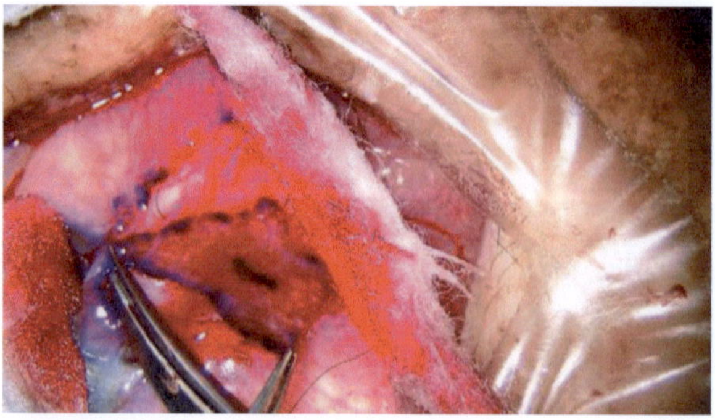

Fig. 6.59 Mark the center of the superficial conjunctival flap and cut the superficial conjunctiva at the corneal limbus

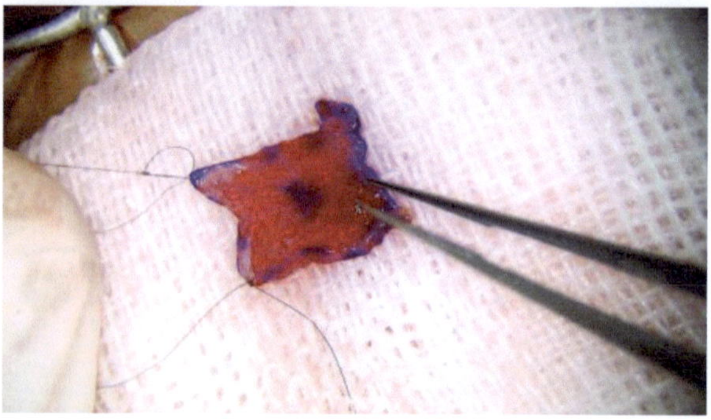

Fig. 6.60 Place the free superficial conjunctival flap on a wet saline gauze and clean up the residual fascia

4. Pterygium excision: Excise the exposed pterygium after removal of the superficial bulbar conjunctiva. Lift the bulbar conjunctiva at the incision of the implant bed with toothed forceps, and separate the conjunctiva from the lower fascia, 1 mm above and below, and 2 mm inside the incision of the lacrimal caruncle conjunctiva. Penetrate the microscissors under the fascia of the upper pterygium body and separate along the scleral surface. Then sever the upper and lower fascia after separation.

   Make a scratch on the pterygium head along the corneal surface to the depth of corneal epithelial layer with closed ophthalmic microscissors, clamp the pterygium head with a toothed forceps, and then exfoliate it along the corneal surface to the neck with microscissors. Next, clamp the pterygium head with a toothed forceps again, and bluntly exfoliate the neck of pterygium with closed microscissors the pterygium is completely dissociated from the corneal surface and limbus, at which time, its three surfaces have been completely disassociated. Clamp the head of pterygium with a toothed forceps to make it fully exposure under a certain tension, and excise the pterygium in the lacrimal caruncle above the terminus of medial rectus with microscissors (Figs. 6.61, 6.62, and 6.63).
5. Wound hemostasis: See Part I of this chapter for related content (Fig. 6.10).
6. 180° transposition of superficial conjunctival flap and suture of autograft: Take the conjunctival autograft from the folded saline-soaked gauze, and transfer it to the exposed sclera after 180° transposition; transpose the lacrimal caruncle side

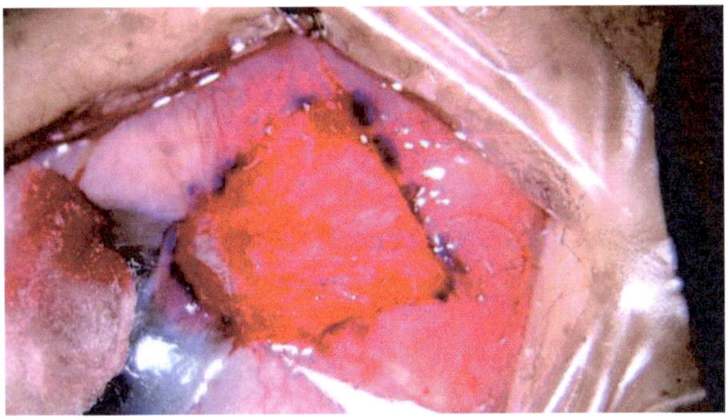

Fig. 6.61 Exposed pterygium after excision of the superficial conjunctiva

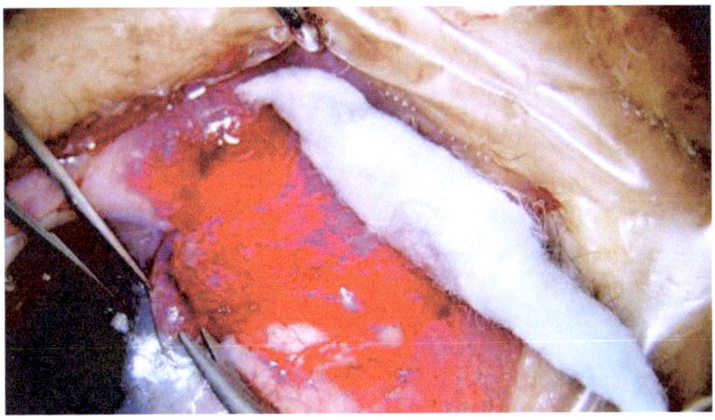

Fig. 6.62 Separate the surrounding bulbar conjunctiva and dissect the pterygium from the head part of the pterygium

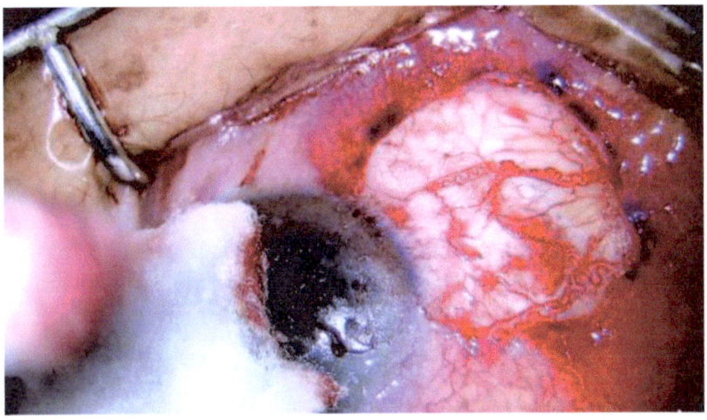

Fig. 6.63 The exposed pterygium is completely excised

of the superficial bulbar conjunctival flap (with marked suture) to the limbal side, and vice versa, with the epithelial surface facing upward. Fix the superficial bulbar conjunctiva of the lacrimal caruncle side to the upper and lower margins of corneal limbus, and the superficial bulbar conjunctiva of the corneal limbus side to the upper and lower margins of sclera in the lacrimal caruncle region by contraposition suture for two stitches each, which should be sutured along with superficial sclera as well. Suture the superior and inferior bulbar conjunctiva with 10-0 nylon thread interruptedly or continuously, and make sure that the superficial bulbar conjunctiva in the lacrimal caruncle is anastomosed end-to-end with its graft bed. A 5–10 mm long thread should be retained to reduce foreign body sensation or sharp pain. The graft suture requirements are as follows:

(a) The four corners should be firmed sutured with the superficial sclera for four stitches.
(b) The graft should be fixed in a tent shape with tension.
(c) The graft should be firmly attached and completely cover the scleral wound.
(d) The transposed conjunctiva graft should be end-to-end anastomosed with its graft bed.
(e) The fascia below the anastomosis should be completely removed.
(f) Continuous suturing of the conjunctiva on the lacrimal caruncle side can prevent the conjunctival flap at the anastomosis from splitting due to ocular mobility (Figs. 6.64, 6.65, and 6.66).

7. Check: After suturing, rinse the surgical area with normal saline, and check for hematoma in the lacrimal caruncle area, aligned joint of the transposed conjunctival flap, active bleeding under the graft, smooth attachment of the transposed conjunctiva to the sclera, and recovery of ocular mobility, etc. Gently squeeze the graft with a medical sponge or cotton swab to remove the hematocele and

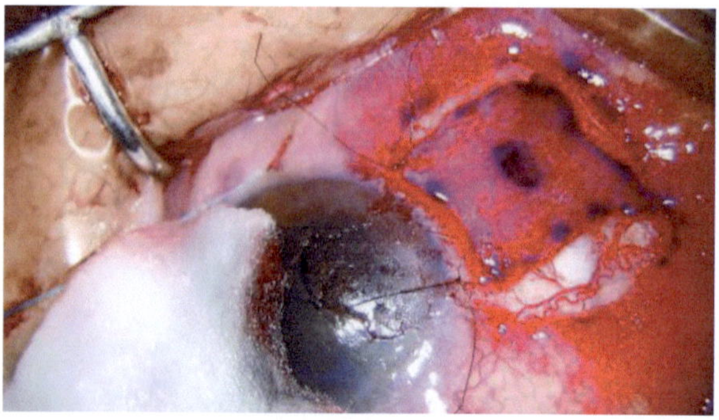

Fig. 6.64 The superficial conjunctival flap is placed back to the scleral wound after transposition 180°, the conjunctival flap lacrimal caruncle side is transposed to the corneal limbus, and the corneal limbus side is transposed to the lacrimal caruncle, the implant is flattened and the mark is confirmed to be on the epithelial surface

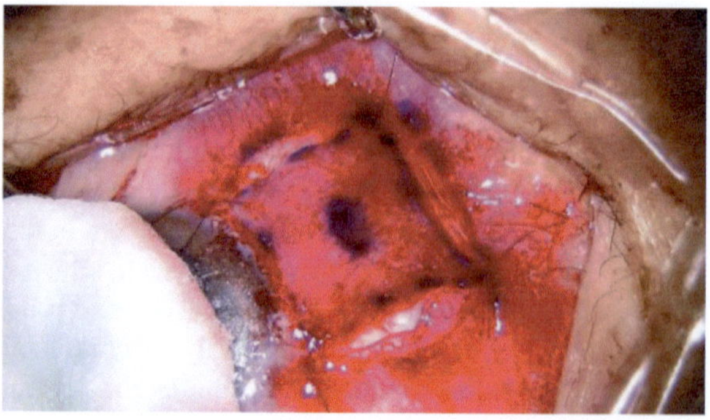

Fig. 6.65 Four corners with superficial sclera are fixed through four sutures, superficial bulbar conjunctival flap is fixed to the scleral wound like a tent shape

effusion under the conjunctival flap, enabling the transposed bulbar conjunctiva flap to tightly adhere to the sclera.

8. Management of corneal surface wound: Wear bandage lenses or cover the corneal bare wound with a bioamnion for protection and pain relief after surgery (Figs. 6.67, 6.68, 6.69, 6.70, 6.71, 6.72 and 6.73).

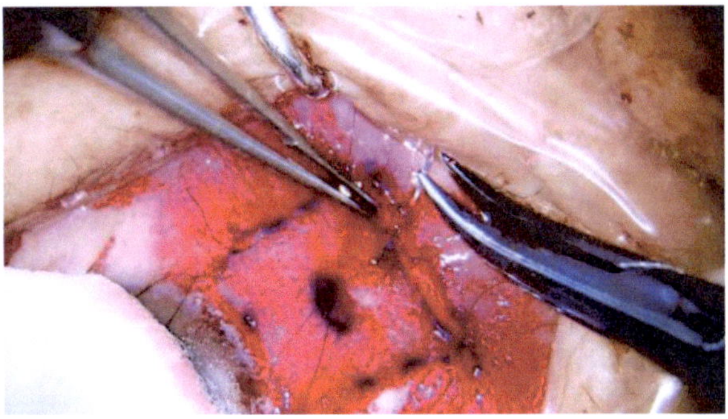

Fig. 6.66 The implant and implant bed bulbar conjunctiva are sutured in end-to-end manner, without superficial sclera involved

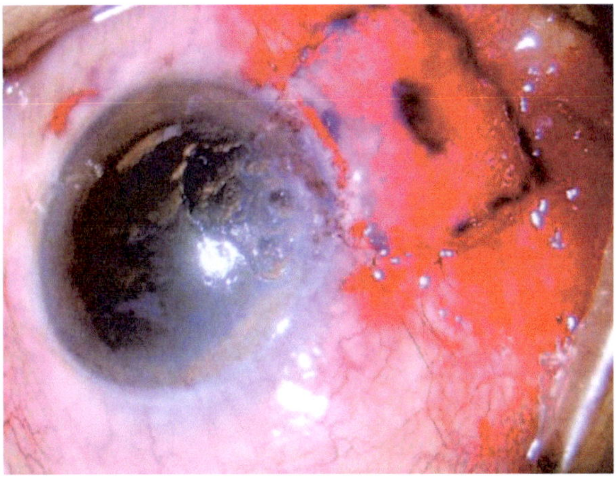

Fig. 6.67 The bulbar conjunctiva of the upper, lower, lacrimal caruncle sides is continuously sutured, and the length of the thread knot is about 10–15 mm

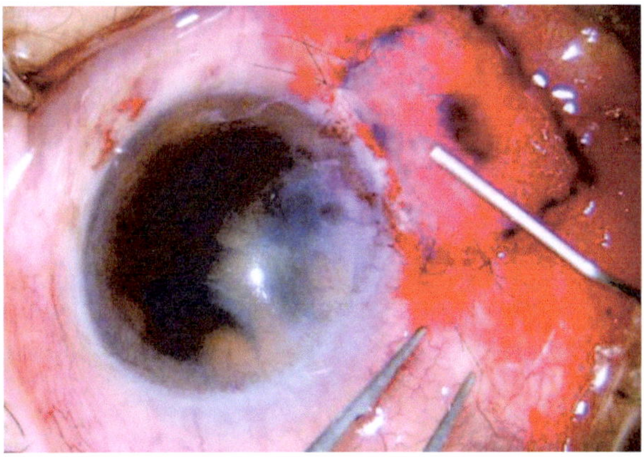

Fig. 6.68 Corneal wound covers bandage lens to relieve pain

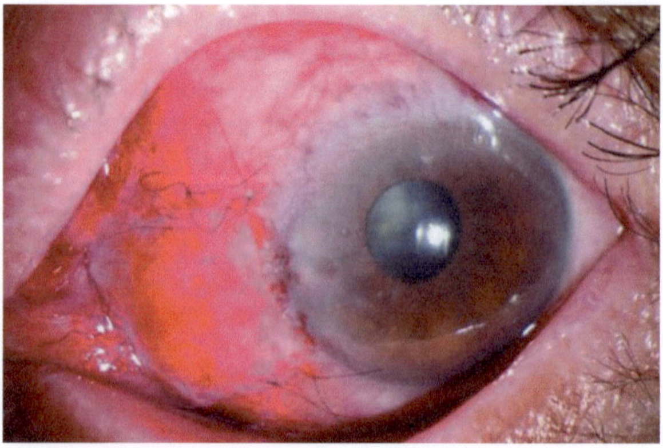
Fig. 6.69 Images on the second day of postoperative, conjunctival flap is flat and well aligned

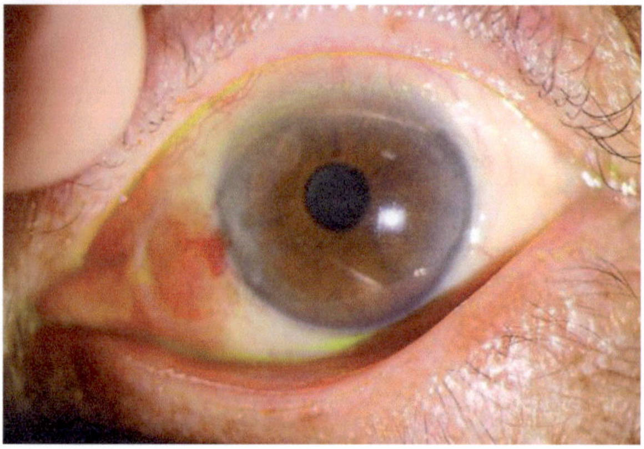
Fig. 6.70 Images at postoperative 3 months

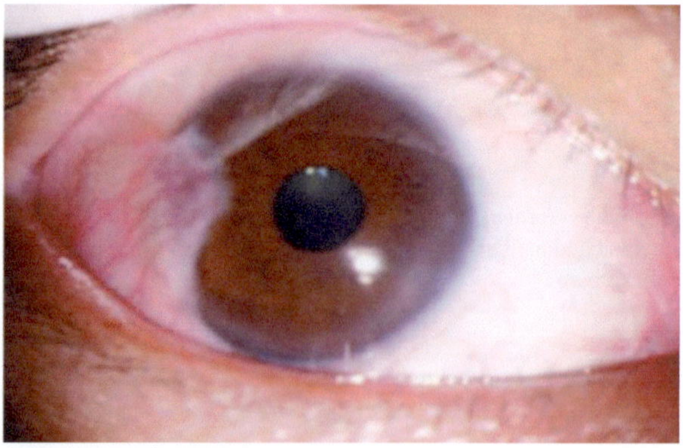
Fig. 6.71 Before CRA

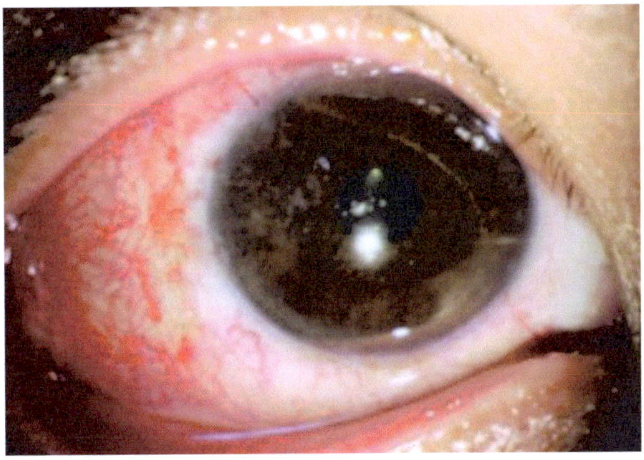

Fig. 6.72 2 weeks after CRA

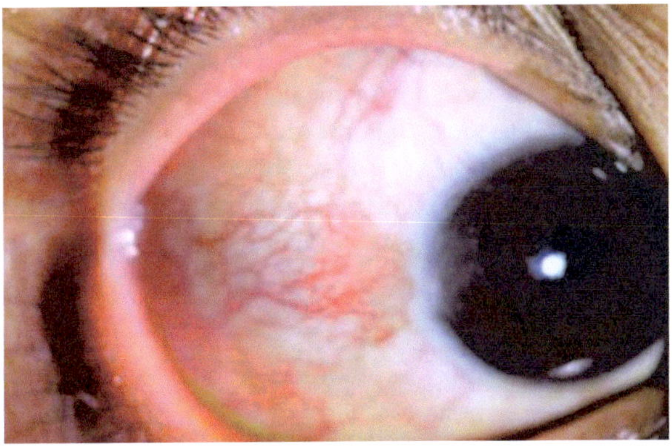

Fig. 6.73 3 months after CRA

6.6 Part VI: Application of Bioglue in Conventional Pterygium Surgery

Medical bioglue is widely used in minimally invasive surgery, obstetrics and gynecology, otorhinolaryngology, and extracorporeal circulation, etc. Porcine fibrin glue is the most common bioglue. The sutures left in the conjunctival sac after pterygium surgery usually lead to foreign body sensation, and some rural patients in remote areas face the difficulty of stitches removal in hospital. To solve these two problems, attempts have been made to use the porcine fibrin glue (i.e., a medical bioglue) to fixedly adhere the bulbar conjunctival graft to the sclera, thereby minimizing or eliminating the use of sutures.

However, bioglues have limited adhesion, and the conjunctival graft may fall off under the friction of long-term blinking, thus exposing the sclera and causing severe complications. Therefore, they should be used with caution for some rural patients in remote areas who cannot seek medical attention in time. In addition, the high cost of bioglue also limits the popularity of this procedure.

6.6.1 Indications

1. Same as those for conventional pterygium excision with free conjunctival flap autograft.
2. Degenerative pterygium.
3. Grade **1** or **2** static pterygium.
4. Pterygium below grade **2** in elderly patients.

6.6.2 Surgical Steps

1. Anesthesia: See Part I of this chapter for related content (see Figs. 6.1 and 6.2).
2. Fixation of eyeballs: See Part I of this chapter for related content (see Fig. 6.3).
3. Pterygium excision: According to the common practice of conventional pterygium excision, draw a conjunctival incision line from 5.5 mm of the corneal limbus to the terminus of medial rectus. The steps for excision of pterygium are identical to those in Part I of this chapter (Figs. 6.74 and 6.75).
4. Wound hemostasis: The scleral wound surface for the transplantation of bulbar conjunctival flap with bioglue should be dry and free from bleeding and exudate. In case of significant vascular hemorrhage, cauterize the bleeding vessels with

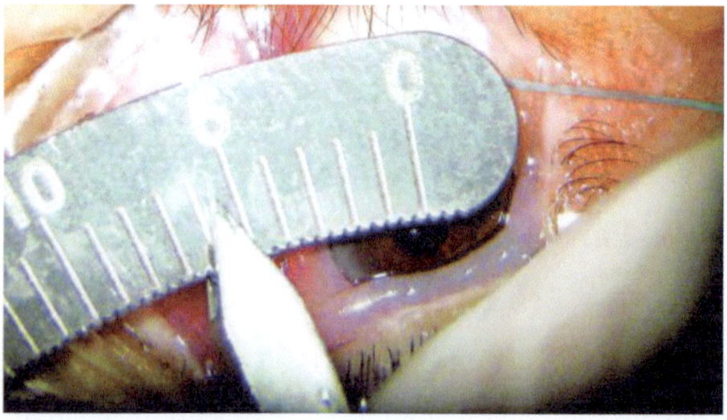

Fig. 6.74 The pterygium incision using bioglue is 5.5 mm and reaches the end of the medial rectus muscle

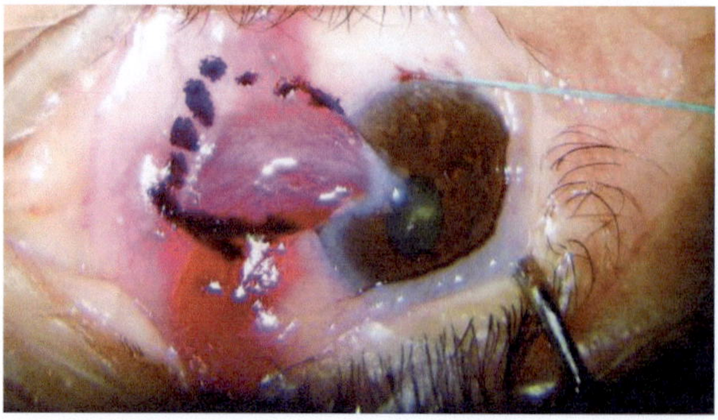

Fig. 6.75 The extent of pterygium excision is labeled using a marker pen

an ophthalmo bipolar or electrocoagulation hemostat; in case of mild errhysis, the dry/wet cotton pads for compressing the exposed scleral surface can be replaced twice or above (Fig. 6.76).

5. Preparation of superiorly free bulbar conjunctival autograft: Release the eyeball traction wire and instruct the patient to look down (the wire should be guided downward by an assistant if patients can hardly cooperate). Where a bioglue is used to attach the grafted globular conjunctiva flap, the upper bulbar conjunctiva should be 0.5 mm larger than the wound surface to reduce the tension between the autograft and the graft bed during adhesion. Other requirements and procedures are the same as those in Part I of this chapter. Move the superior free bulbar conjunctival flap to the corneal wound surface, with its fascia facing upward, and lay it flat on the corneal wound surface with the corneal limbus aligned; wait until the surgical area is completely dry (Figs. 6.77 and 6.78).
6. Cleaning of scleral exposed surface: Clean the wound bleeding in the surgical area with an absorbent sponge, resettle the graft bed of bulbar conjunctiva, and confirm that the scleral wound surface is dry and clean.
7. Adhesion of free bulbar conjunctival autograft with bioglue: Apply a small amount of bioglue to the scleral exposed surface (or omit this step); disassociate

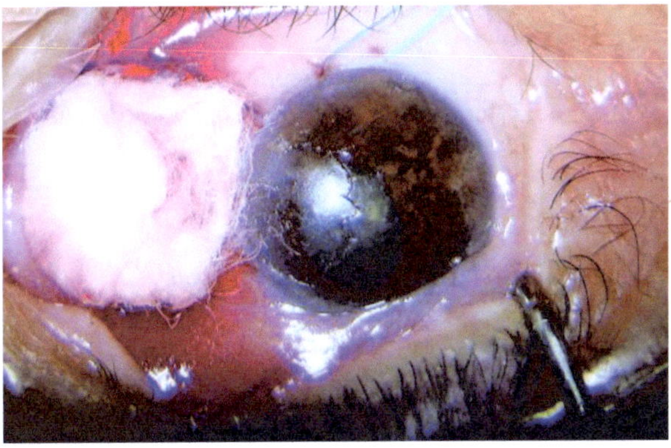

Fig. 6.76 After pterygium excision, the scleral wound is compressed and dried with two cotton blocks, dry and wet alternatively

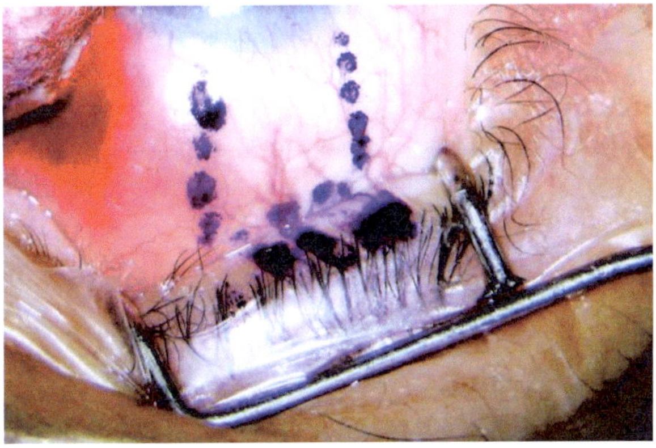

Fig. 6.77 The upper implant sampling area is 0.5 mm larger than the implant bed to avoid binding difficulties

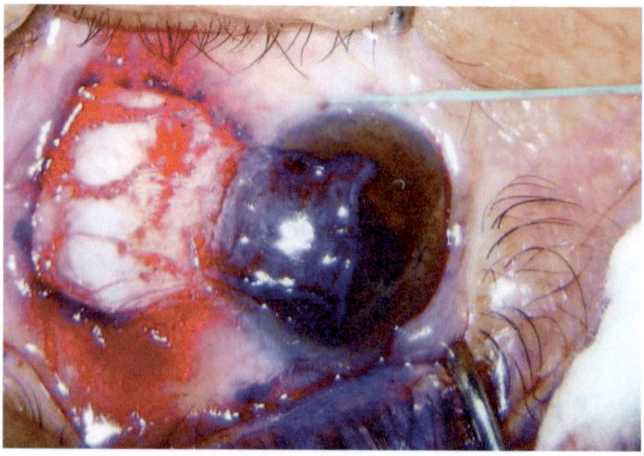

Fig. 6.78 The conjunctival flap is placed on the corneal wound with the fascial side facing up, the corneal limbus is aligned with the corneal limbus, waiting for the scleral wound to dry

the free bulbar conjunctiva autograft from the corneal wound surface, move it to the exposed sclera with a toothed microforceps, and stick it to the sclera in the surgical area with its fascia facing downward, the bulbar conjunctiva on the corneal limbus side of the autograft opposite to the graft bed of corneal limbus, and the bulbar conjunctiva in the fornix area above the autograft opposite to the bulbar conjunctiva in the lacrimal caruncle of the graft bed; press the autograft lightly with an absorbent sponge to make it adhere to the scleral surface via bioglue. Intermittently suture the superior and inferior bulbar conjunctiva on the corneal limbus for one stitch each, as well as on the lacrimal caruncle side for one stitch each. Firmly suture the four corners with the superficial sclera for four stitches.

Fill the anastomosis between the graft bed and the bulbar conjunctiva autograft with bioglue, and clamp double ends of bulbar conjunctiva tightly with a toothed microforceps for about 1 min to ensure firm adherence. Patiently inject bioglue by segments for the tripartite graft and the graft bed of bulbar conjunctiva, and clamp the joint for a while to ensure firm adherence. Grafting requirements are as follows:

(a) The four corners should be firmed sutured with the superficial sclera for four stitches.
(b) The bulbar conjunctiva graft should be 0.5 mm larger than the graft bed to reduce tension.
(c) The graft should be firmly attached and completely cover the scleral wound.
(d) The conjunctiva graft and its graft bed should be bonded end to end without gaps.
(e) The conjunctival and scleral surfaces should be free of errhysis and exudation.
(f) Once confirming that the graft is firmly adhered to the graft bed, it should wait for 2–3 min until the wound surface is dry (Figs. 6.79, 6.80, 6.81, 6.82, and 6.83).

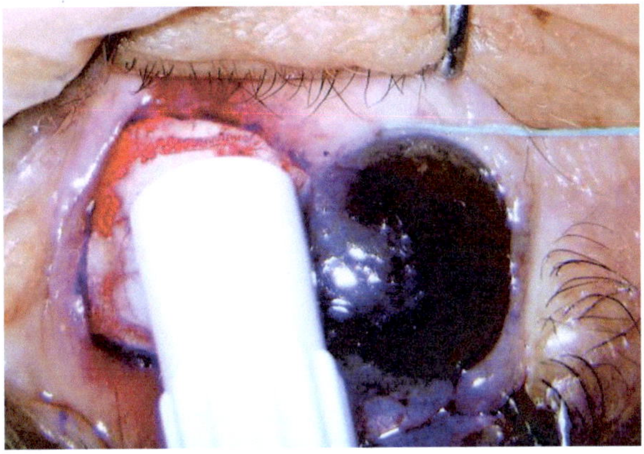

Fig. 6.79 Inject a small amount of bioglue into the scleral wound

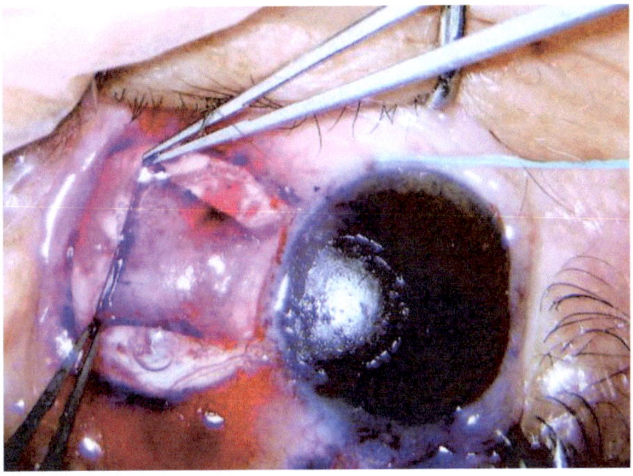

Fig. 6.80 After injecting bioglue into the scleral surface, the implant is flipped and flattened, or the conjunctival flap can be flipped and flattened directly without bioglue injection

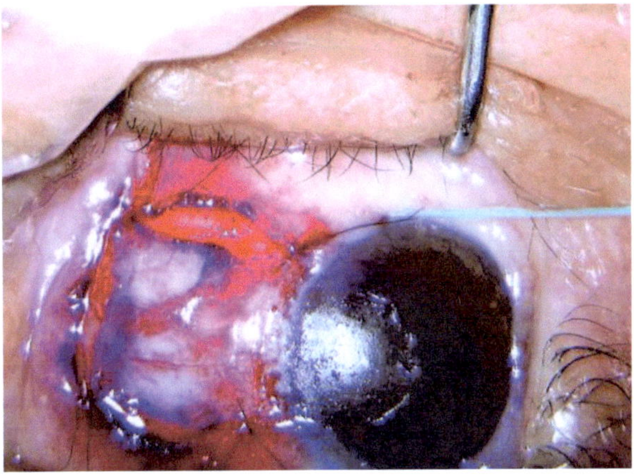

Fig. 6.81 10-0 nylon thread is used to fix the implant with four sutures (with superficial sclera)

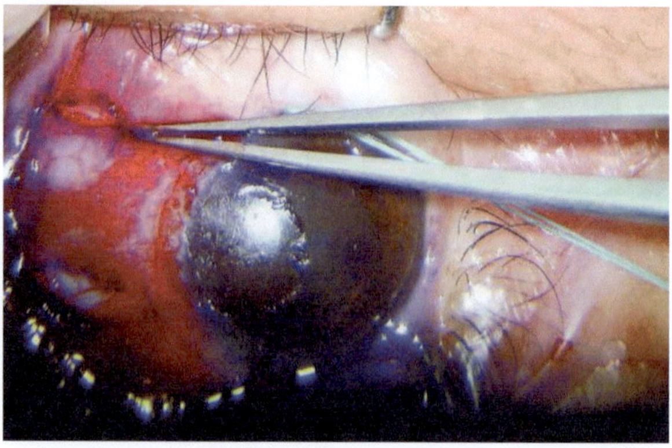

Fig. 6.82 Inject bioglue into the anastomostosis, patiently clamp the implant and the implant bed bulbar conjunctiva for firm binding, and inject bioglue + clamping by segment until they are completely binding

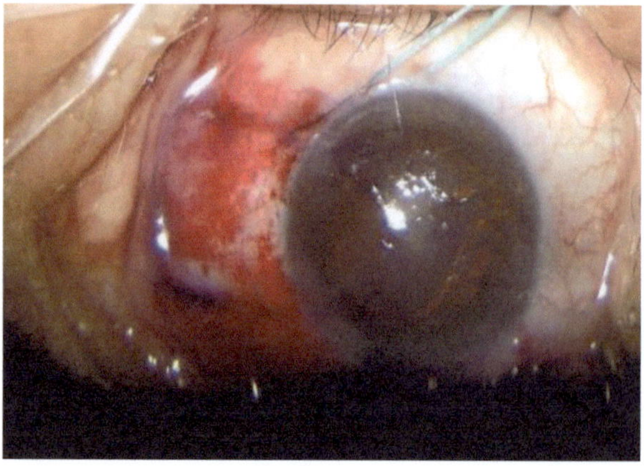

Fig. 6.83 The tripartite implant is firmly binding with the conjunctiva of the implant bed

8. Check: After adhesion, it is necessary to check whether the bulbar conjunctiva at the anastomotic site is jointed neatly, whether there is active bleeding flap under the conjunctiva, and whether the adhesion with bioglue is reliable. This procedure does not require rinsing any wound with normal saline, in case of damage to the adhesive force of bioglue. After surgery, the bulbar conjunctiva on the scleral surface should be gently pressed again with an absorbent sponge to confirm reliable adhesion of the graft.
9. Management of corneal wound surface: Wear corneal bandage lenses to protect the postoperative bare wound and relieve pain. A pressure bandage should be applied to the wound for 24 h after surgery to ensure reliable adhesion of bioglue (Figs. 6.84 and 6.85).

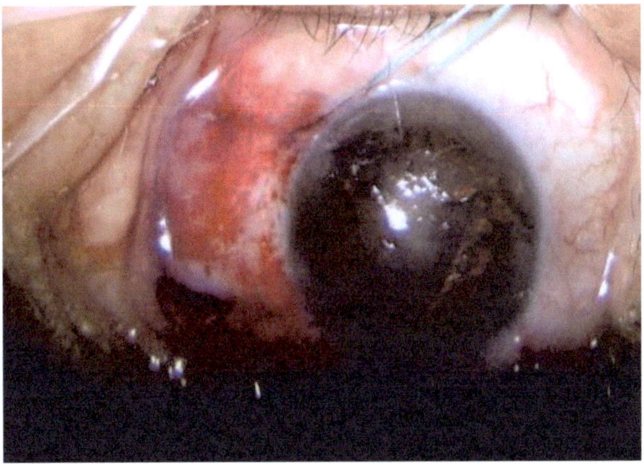

Fig. 6.84 Images on the second day of postoperative, conjunctival flap is flat and bandage lend is place properly

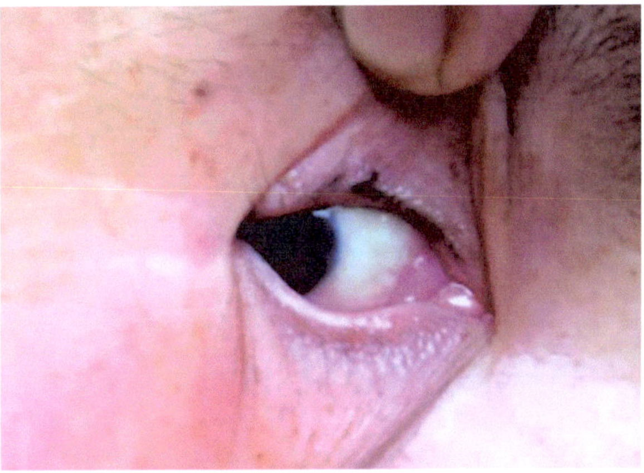

Fig. 6.85 Images of the patient taken by the family member using a phone at postoperative 2 months, aesthetic grading is Grade 2

References

1. Fengming L, Lixin X. Chinese ophthalmology. 3rd ed. Beijing: People's Medical Publishing House; 2014. p. 1250–5.
2. Cornelius CR. Recurrence rate and complications of pterygium extended removal followed by extended conjunctival transplant. Cornea. 2017;36(1):101103.
3. Hirst LW. Recurrence and complications after 1000 surgeries using pterygium extended removal followed by extended conjunctival transplant. Ophthalmology. 2012;119(11):22052210.
4. Jap A, Chan C, Lim L, et al. Conjunctival rotation autograft for pterygium. An alternative to conjunctival autografting. Ophthalmology. 1999;106(1):6771.

Chapter 7
Recurrent Pterygium Surgery

Kehua Wang and Congxiang Wang

7.1 Part I: Overview of Recurrent Pterygium

Recurrent pterygium refers to pterygium recurrence following resection operation of primary pterygium. Recurrent pterygium, which differs pathologically from primary pterygium, is a fibrous vascular tissue growing on the cornea without elastic degeneration. It mainly infiltrates the superficial sclera and Tenon's capsule downward and invades the corneal stroma to firmly adhere to the underlying tissue [1].

Recurrent pterygium may impose restrictions on ocular motility due to scar tissue or invasion of horizontal muscle sheath, causing diplopia and ocular motility disorders, and even blindness in severe cases.

7.1.1 Etiology of Recurrent Pterygium

1. Preoperative etiology: (1) poor control of ocular surface inflammation, in case of severe preoperative congestion due to pterygium, well-controlled inflammation is required before operation; (2) blepharitis, eyelash follicle mites, severe meibomain gland dysfunction (MGD), which may increase the risk of postoperative recurrence of pterygium; (3) a high recurrence rate in young people and those with a familial genetic predisposition to pterygium.
2. Intraoperative etiology: (1) inadequate lesion resection; (2) crude surgical instruments: in the absence of microscopic ophthalmic surgery, the instruments and

K. Wang (✉) · C. Wang
Changsha Aier Eye Hospital, Changsha, China

C. Wang, S. Li (eds.), *Pterygium Surgery*,
https://doi.org/10.1007/978-981-99-6843-5_7

needles used are crude; (3) improper surgical procedures: e.g., simple excision and pterygium head transposition; (4) failure in complete excision of subconjunctival fascia tissue adjacent to pterygium due to insufficient intraoperative experience.

3. Postoperative etiology: (1) poor control of early postoperative inflammation; (2) lack of medical attention to xerophthalmia due to poor sleep; (3) familial inheritance; (4) ethnic difference; (5) postoperative overexposure to UV.

7.1.2 *Principles of Recurrent Pterygium Surgery*

Surgery, as the only treatment for recurrent pterygium, shall be performed after meeting the following principles: (1) adequate control of ocular surface inflammation; (2) an interval of at least half year from the latest pterygium operation; (3) appropriate surgical procedures depending on difficulty; (4) operation by experienced and qualified surgeons.

7.2 Part II: Surgical Procedures of Recurrent Pterygium

The choice of surgical procedures for recurrent pterygium mainly depends on the following four points:

1. Scope, location and depth of symblepharon.
2. Extent of lacrimal caruncle displacement.
3. Depth and location of corneal stroma invasion.
4. Structural integrity of the superior or inferior bulbar conjunctiva.

Surgical procedures are determined according to the above four points. Lamellar keratoplasty is required for scar access to the deep corneal stroma (excluding corneal degeneration) or to the deep pupillary stroma. The followings are three common procedures for treating recurrent pterygium in the author's hospital:

7.2.1 *Recurrent Pterygium Excision + Autogenous Free Conjunctival Flap Transplantation + Bioamnion Covering [2]*

It's indicated to recurrent pterygium with superficial symblepharon, limited scope and superficial involvement of corneal stroma, also known as "trilogy for recurrent pterygium" (Fig. 7.1).

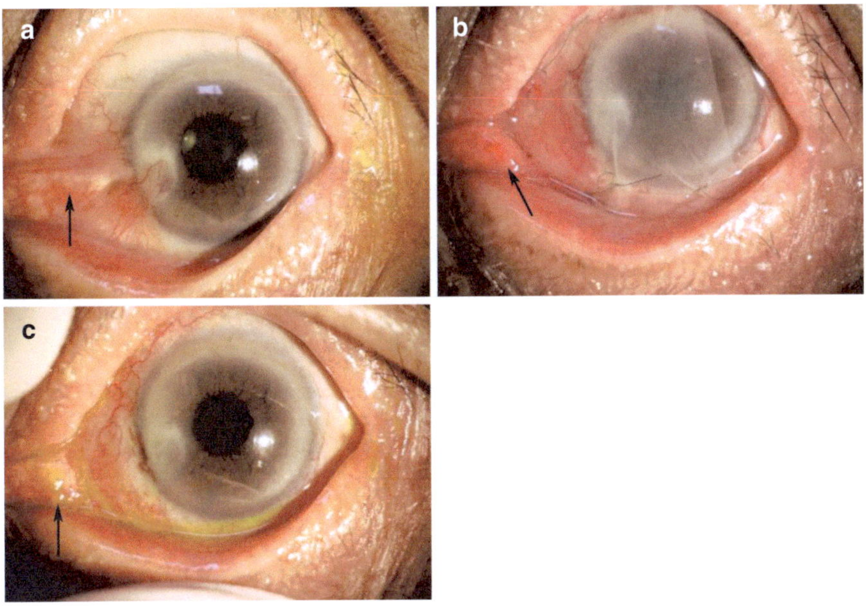

Fig. 7.1 Pre- and postoperative status of trilogy. (**a**) Preoperatively, moderate recurrent pterygium with mild symblepharon and pure local degeneration of corneal stroma and without involvement of deep corneal stroma; (**b**) on POD2, well-placed bioamnion and good reattachment of lacrimal caruncle; (**c**) review on POW2; black arrows in (**a**–**c**) show changes in pre- and postoperative locations of lacrimal caruncle

Trilogy may also be performed in case of severe recurrent pterygium with scars in superficial corneal stroma, absence of scars in the pupillary region, or scars in the superficial pupillary region, superior or inferior bulbar conjunctiva with normal color and complete structure, and reattachment of lacrimal caruncle following the relief of symblepharon (Figs. 7.2 and 7.3).

7.2.2 Recurrent Pterygium Excision + Fresh Bioamnion Graft + Autotransplantation of Free Conjunctival Flap + Bioamnion Covering [3]

For any recurrent pterygium larger than one quadrant or any scleral wound scar larger than four clocks, scleral lesions need to be managed. A layer of fresh bioamnion applied to the wound after scleral cicatrectomy can accelerate its repair. Recurrent pterygium excision + fresh bioamnion graft + autotransplantation of free conjunctival flap + bioamnion covering (also known as recurrent pterygium tetralogy) can better manage patients with large-area scleral scars.

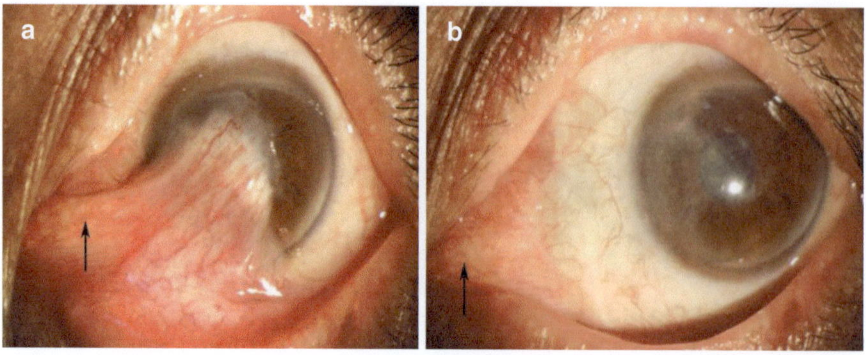

Fig. 7.2 Pre- and postoperative status of trilogy for recurrent pterygium. (**a**) Preoperatively, severe recurrent pterygium, whose head covered the pupils, accompanied by transposition of lacrimal caruncle, symblepharon and ocular motility disorders, was the first relapse, manifested with shallow scars on anterior segment OCT, and proposed to be treated by "trilogy or lamellar keratoplasty for recurrent pterygium"; (**b**) trilogy for recurrent pterygium was proposed due to the intraoperative findings of minor corneal involvement, prominent by involvement of superficial pupillary stroma; the photos on POM2 revealed relief of symblepharon, good reattachment of lacrimal caruncle, normal ocular motility, and recovery of visual acuity to 0.8; black arrows indicated changes in pre- and postoperative locations of lacrimal caruncle

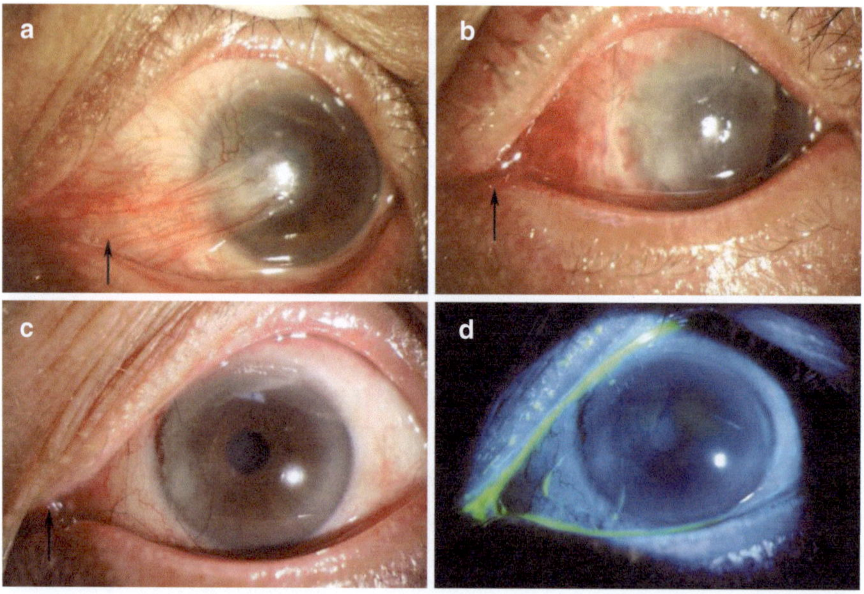

Fig. 7.3 Pre- and postoperative status of trilogy for recurrent pterygium. (**a**) Preoperatively, severe recurrent pterygium covered the pupils, accompanied by minor adhesion and superficial scars; (**b**) on POD2, reattachment of lacrimal caruncle, corneal wounds covered by bioamnion and localized degeneration of peripheral cornea with little effect on visual acuity in the pupillary area were observed; (**c**) at the time of stitches removal on POD10, the dissolved bioamnion and well-recovered corneal wounds were seen; (**d**) no fluorescein staining (negative) was found in cornea and conjunctiva; black arrows in (**a–c**) indicated changes in pre- and postoperative locations of lacrimal caruncle

Due to its complexity and difficulty, the tetralogy requires patience particularly when managing scleral scars and should be performed by an experienced specialist in ocular surface surgery (see the surgical procedures in this Part for pictures).

7.2.3 Recurrent Pterygium Excision + Autotransplantation of Free Conjunctival Flap + Lamellar Keratoplasty

Lamellar keratoplasty is required in case of recurrent pterygium with severe symblepharon, transposition and deformity of lacrimal caruncle, and invasion of 1/2 corneal thickness by stromal scars, or scars located in deep pupillary stroma (Fig. 7.4).

Whether recurrent pterygium excision + autotransplantation of free conjunctival flap + bioamnion covering can solve ocular motility disorders should be assessed if the eyeballs are attached to eyelids due to severe symblepharon or multiple operations for pterygium lead to local scars invading 1/2 or above of the corneal thickness. If the conclusion was negative, a corneal marginal lamellar keratoplasty

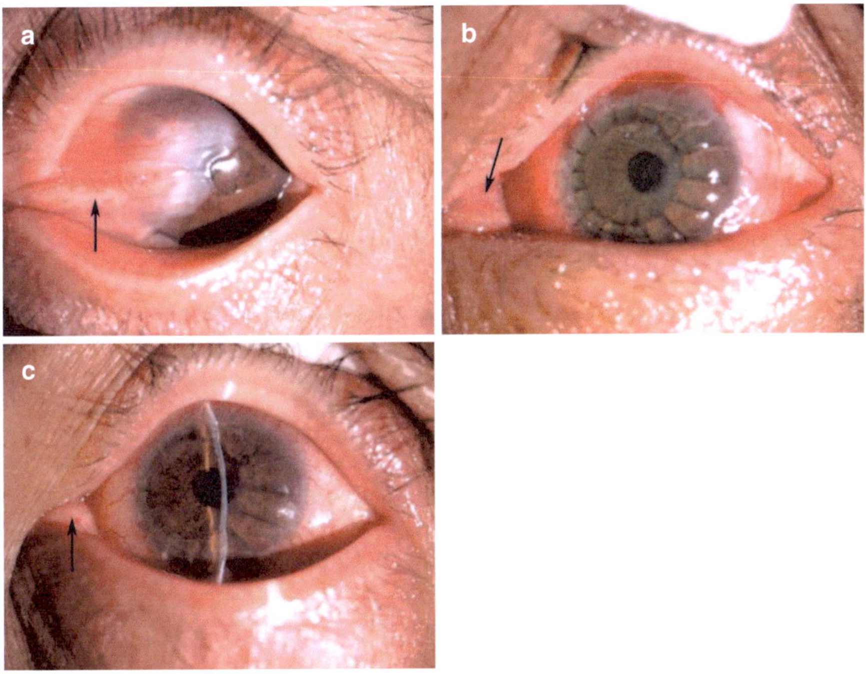

Fig. 7.4 Therapeutic effect of giant recurrent pterygium. (**a**) Preoperatively, the recurrent pterygium covered the pupils, with the invasion of scars into deep corneal stroma of pupillary region, severe symblepharon, transposition and deformity of lacrimal caruncle, ocular motility disorders and visual acuity under manual operation; (**b**) on POD2, reattachment of lacrimal caruncle, relief of symblepharon, normal ocular motility and uncorrected visual acuity (UCVA) of 0.25 were found; (**c**) on POW2, the UCVA of 0.4 was detected; black arrows in (**a–c**) indicated changes in pre- and postoperative locations of lacrimal caruncle

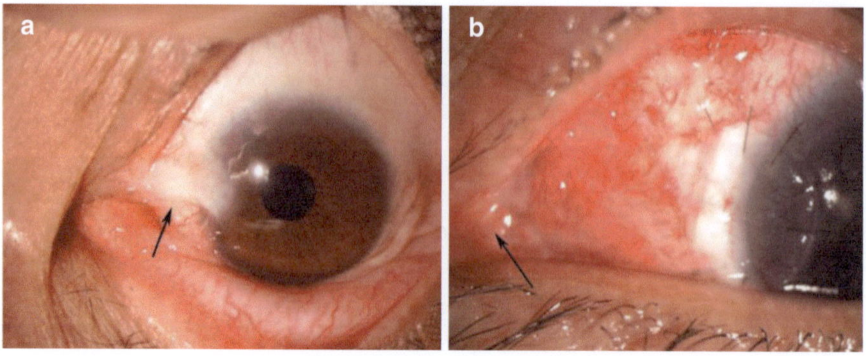

Fig. 7.5 Therapeutic effect of recurrent pterygium following multiple excisions. (**a**) Following four times of excision and recurrence locally, the pterygium in the left eye adhered to the nasal eyelids, with scar invasion into the deep corneal stroma, severe diplopia, and attachment of eyeballs to lacrimal caruncle, attachment of displaced lacrimal caruncle to the palpebral fissure due to scar adhesion, so that the patient could not work normally and suffered a lot; (**b**) after the conjunctival suture was removed on POD7 of recurrent pterygium excision + lysis of scars + crescentic lamellar keratoplasty + autotransplantation of free conjunctival flap, relieved symblepharon, good reattachment of lacrimal caruncle, and free mobility of eyeballs were observed; black arrows in (**a**, **b**) indicated changes in pre- and postoperative locations of lacrimal caruncle

is required to relieve the pain of diplopia and ocular motility disorders, even if the recurrent pterygium fails to invade the pupillary zone (Fig. 7.5).

7.3 Part III: Surgical Steps for Recurrent Pterygium

7.3.1 Surgical Steps of Recurrent Pterygium Excision + Autotransplantation of Free Conjunctival Flap + Bioamnion Covering

1. Indications: This procedure is indicated to recurrent pterygium with non-autologous transplantation of conjunctival flap in the primary surgery, intact superior or inferior conjunctiva and minor symblepharon. Preoperative anterior segment OCT is required, indicating that indicating that the lesion has not yet invaded the deep corneal stroma.
2. Surgical steps The surgical steps are as follows:
    (a) Anesthesia: See Part I of Chap. 6 for related content (see Figs. 6.1 and 6.2).
    (b) Fixation of eyeballs: See Part I of Chap. 6 for related content (see Fig. 6.3).
    (c) Recurrent pterygium excision: Different from primary pterygium, recurrent pterygium is firmly adhered to corneal stroma, superficial sclera and fascia, so its excision needs patience and care. First, excise the head of recurrent pterygium parallel to the cornea arc (or cut the adhesive band directly from

the corneal limbus); then totally resect and release the scleral adhesion band parallel to the scleral surface, while protecting the sclera tissue and avoiding damage to the deep stroma. If any scar deeply invaded the sclera, part of it on the superficial scleral surface may be retained but the wound surface should be smooth. The surgery should cover the normal Tenon's capsule in the nasal lacrimal caruncle to make it completely reattached. Clean the corneal and scleral wounds. No treatment is required for peripheral corneal degeneration that does not affect visual acuity (Figs. 7.6, 7.7, and 7.8).

(d) Reattachment of lacrimal caruncle: The recurrent pterygium-associated scars tend to pull the bulbar conjunctiva in the lacrimal caruncle region to the corneal surface, causing symblepharon and ocular motility disorders, and affecting tear circulation; therefore, a critical step in surgery for recurrent pterygium is to restore the involved lacrimal caruncle to its normal position. Clear all residual tissue in the corneal and scleral surgical areas to

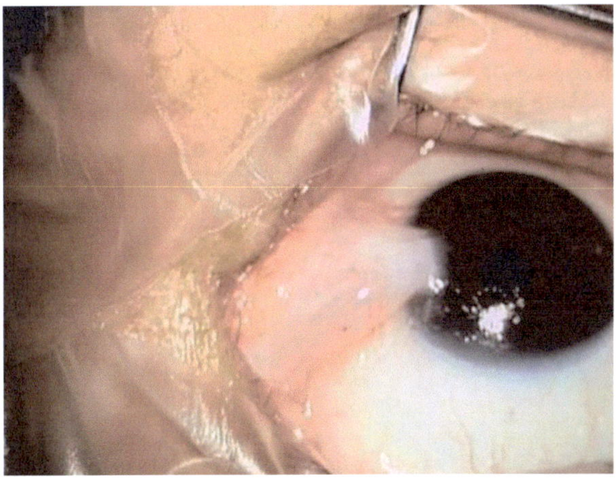

Fig. 7.6 Moderate recurrent pterygium without deep scarring, without severe symblepharon, with intact superior bulbar conjunctiva, triple surgery for recurrent pterygium is allowed

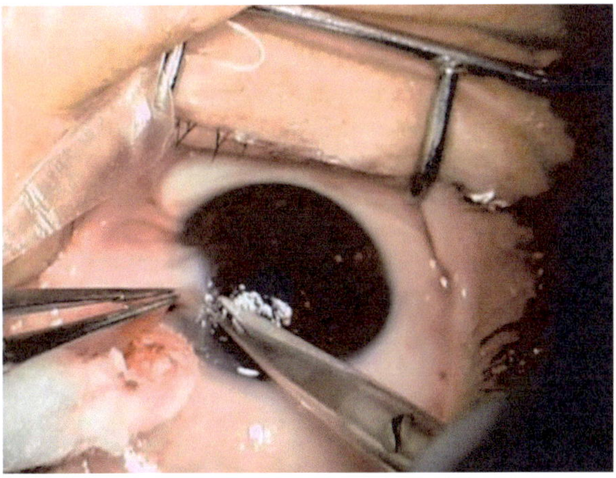

Fig. 7.7 During the surgery, firstly dissect the head and patiently separate the corneal contour

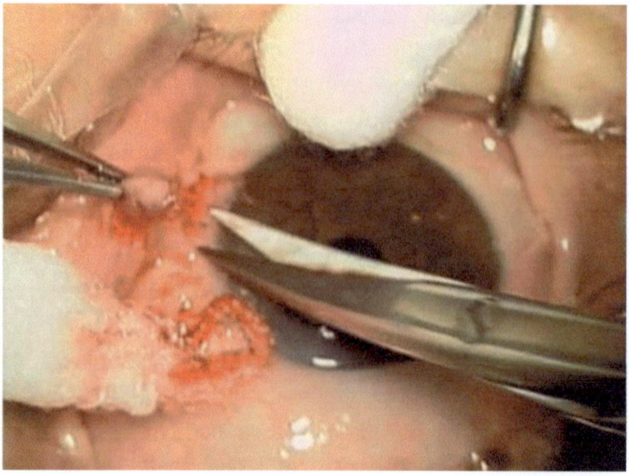

Fig. 7.8 Remove the scar at the operating field in parallel to scleral surface and separate until the sublacrimal Tenon's cyst

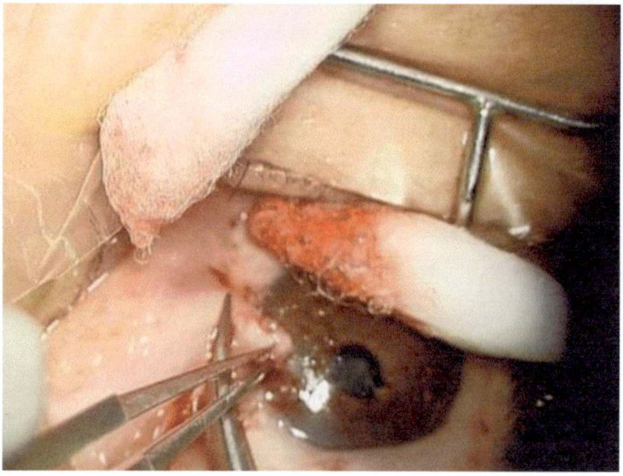

Fig. 7.9 Reset the lacrimal caruncle, cut the recurrent pterygium scar in front of the lacrimal caruncle away from 1.5 mm in front of lacrimal caruncle conjunctiva

confirm whether the symblepharon is completely relieved. Then clamp the cicatrix tissue of recurrent pterygium with a toothed microforceps, and resect the recurrent pterygium and its adherent tissue parallel to the anterior lacrimal caruncle and at a distance of 1.5 mm. Clear the residual scar tissue of corneal and scleral wounds, while protecting the corneal and scleral stroma (Figs. 7.9 and 7.10).

(e) Preparation of free bulbar conjunctival flap and transplantation to the surgical area: the free bulbar conjunctival flap should have the identical size with the surgical area to completely cover the scleral wound (Figs. 7.11 and 7.12).
(f) Coverage of surgical area with bioamnions: corneal and conjunctival wounds are covered with bioamnions to accelerate healing, minimize cicatrization, control inflammatory response, and reduce the recurrence of pterygium (Figs. 7.13 and 7.14).

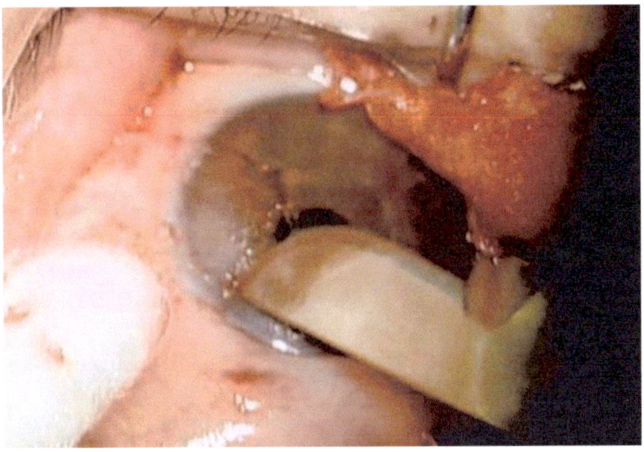

Fig. 7.10 Clean the residual tissues of the cornea and scleral surface operating field, and completely relieve symblepharon

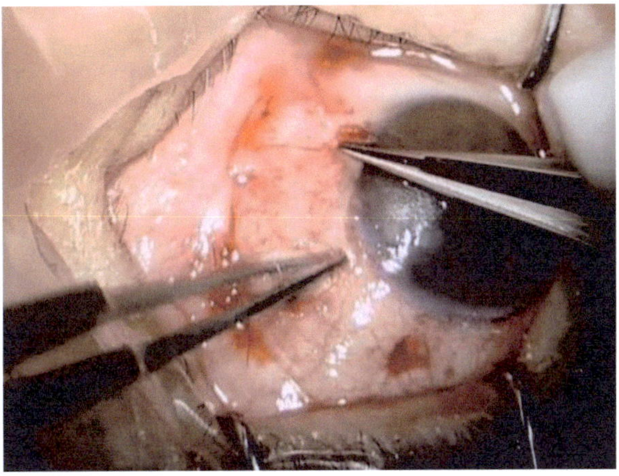

Fig. 7.11 Place the free bulbar conjunctival implant at equal size with the operating field to the operating field

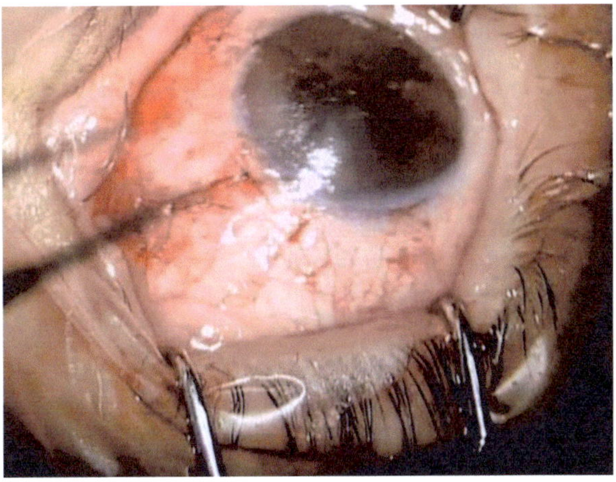

Fig. 7.12 Suture the free bulbar conjunctival flap, at which time the lacrimal caruncle has been reset, the symblepharon has been relived, and the scars of the corneal and scleral wounds have been removed

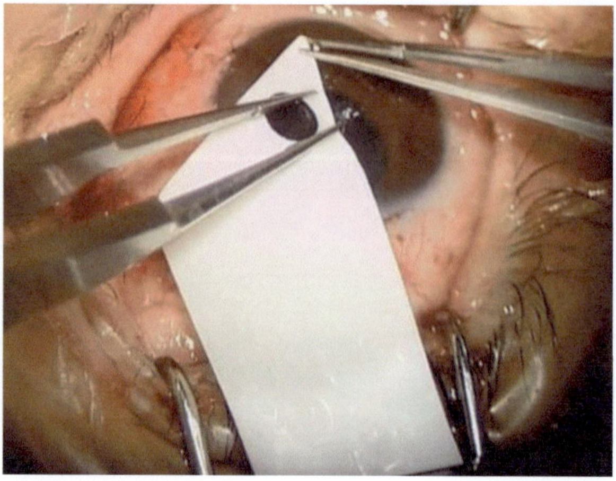

Fig. 7.13 Monolamellar amniotic membrane at 10 mm × 15 mm (monolamellar biological amniotic membrane available in 2013 only)

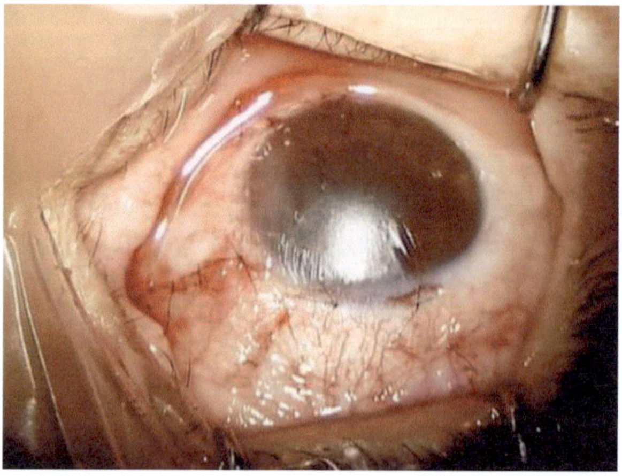

Fig. 7.14 Biological amniotic membrane wraps corneal wound and part of the upper conjunctival wound

(g) Management of superior bulbar conjunctiva: level the superior bioamnion and manage the superior bulbar conjunctiva. For large conjunctival wounds, the bioamnion may be partially sutured to the superior bulbar conjunctiva with 10-0 nylon suture.

(h) Check: rinse the wounds with normal saline, and check for hematoma in the lacrimal caruncle area, good reattachment of lacrimal caruncle, aligned joint of conjunctival flap, active subconjunctival bleeding, smooth attachment of the transplanted conjunctiva to the sclera, tight wrapping of corneal wounds by bioamnions, effusion and hematocele under bioamnions, and recovery of ocular mobility, etc. Gently squeeze the bulbar conjunctival graft and the corneal wound bioamnion with a medical sponge or cotton swab to remove the hematocele and effusion under the conjunctival flap and the bioamnion, enabling the conjunctival flap to tightly adhere to the sclera and the bioamnion to completely cover the corneal wound.

7.3.2 Surgical Steps of Recurrent Pterygium Excision + Fresh Bioamnion Graft + Autotransplantation of Free Conjunctival Flap + Bioamnion Covering

For any recurrent pterygium with adhesion larger than one corneal quadrant or any scleral wound larger than four clocks, the tetralogy for recurrent pterygium can be selected.

The surgical steps are as follows:

1. Anesthesia: See Part I of Chap. 6 for related content (see Figs. 6.1 and 6.2).
2. Fixation of eyeballs: See Part I of Chap. 6 for related content (see Fig. 6.3).
3. Recurrent pterygium excision: similar to the trilogy of recurrent pterygium, in case of severe adhesion, cut the adhesive band from the corneal limbus, patiently resect and release the scars on the scleral surface, while protecting the sclera and lacrimal caruncle tissue (Figs. 7.15, 7.16, 7.17, and 7.18).
4. Reattachment of lacrimal caruncle: same as that of the trilogy of recurrent pterygium.

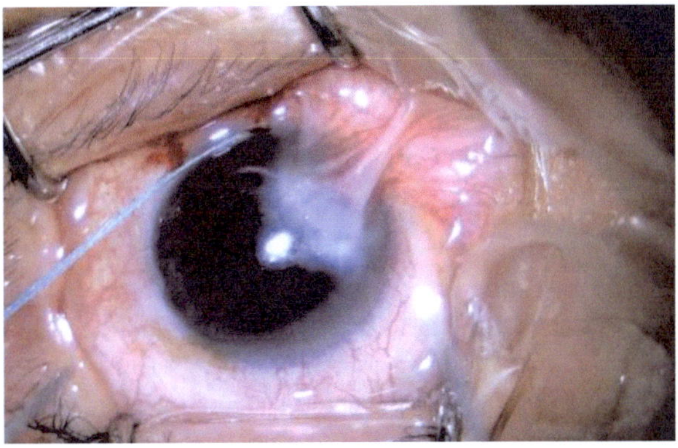

Fig. 7.15 Lesions exceeding 1 corneal quadrant, scleral scarring increasing from 6 points to 11 points, severe symblepharon, and lacrimal caruncle antedisplacement

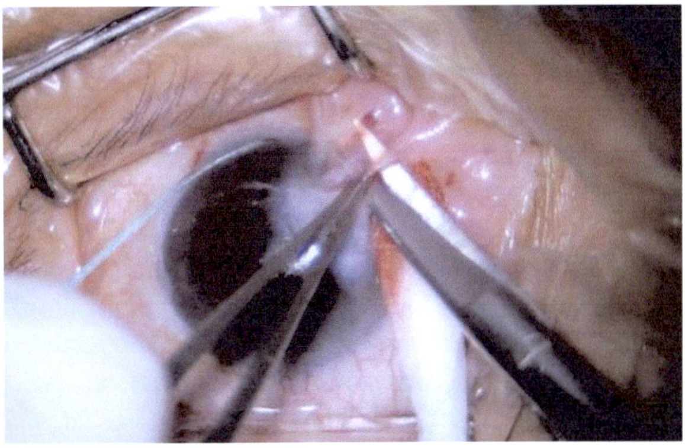

Fig. 7.16 Separate and cut the corneal limbal adhesion tissue

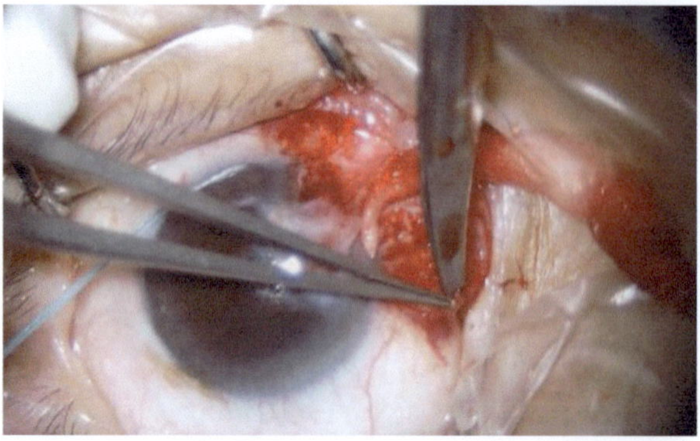

Fig. 7.17 Thoroughly release subconjunctival and scleral surface scars

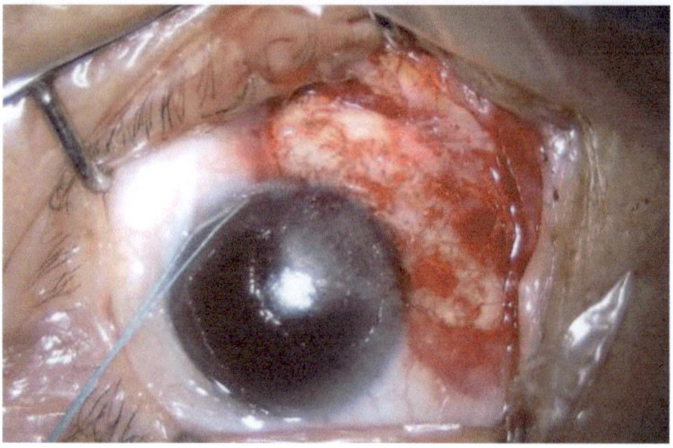

Fig. 7.18 Completely excise recurrent pterygium, scars and adhesion tissue, showing that the conjunctival defect surface is large, and the conventional upper conjunctival flap cannot completely cover the conjunctival defect area

5. Fresh amnion graft: tailor a piece of fresh bioamnion 1 mm larger than the scleral wound, transplant to the scleral wound with its base facing down, and suture it intermittently to the sclera with 100 absorbable sutures. Then insert its edges except for the corneal limbus sided under the adjacent bulbar conjunctiva. This bioamnion is used to protect the scleral wound and serves as a substrate to promote conjunctival epithelization on its surface (Figs. 7.19 and 7.20).
6. Preparation of free bulbar conjunctival flap and transplantation to the surgical area: manage the bulbar conjunctiva and resettle the lacrimal caruncle. Transplant the free bulbar conjunctival flap to the surgical area to cover the fresh bioamnion and anastomose end-to-end with the bulbar conjunctiva of the graft bed. Then suture it for four stitches with the superficial sclera for routine fixation, and allow intermittent or continuous suturing for the rest without the fresh bioamnion (Fig. 7.21).
7. Coverage of corneal wounds with bioamnions: corneal and conjunctival wounds are covered with bioamnions to accelerate healing, minimize cicatrization, control inflammatory response, and reduce the recurrence of pterygium (Fig. 7.22).
8. Management of superior bulbar conjunctiva: level the superior bioamnion and manage the superior bulbar conjunctiva. For large conjunctival wounds, the bio-

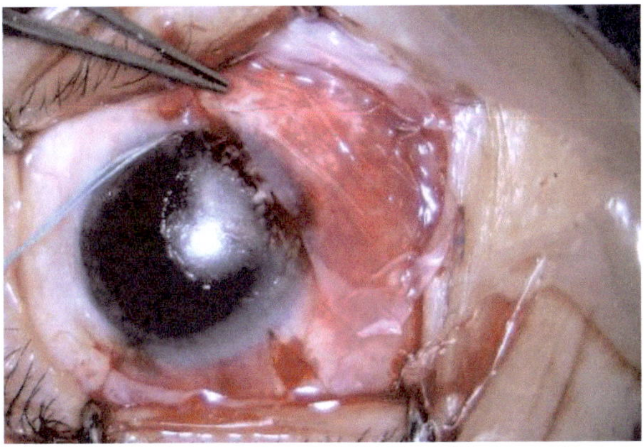

Fig. 7.19 Fresh amniotic membranes are transplanted into the conjunctival wound and inserted below the conjunctival incision

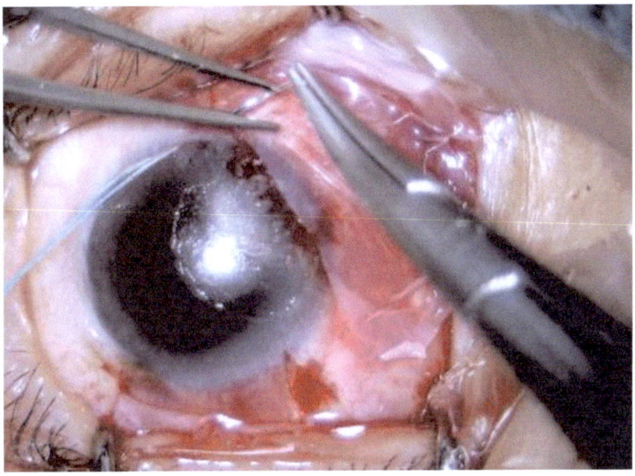

Fig. 7.20 10-0 thread is used to fix fresh amniotic membrane to the scleral wound through intermittent sutures

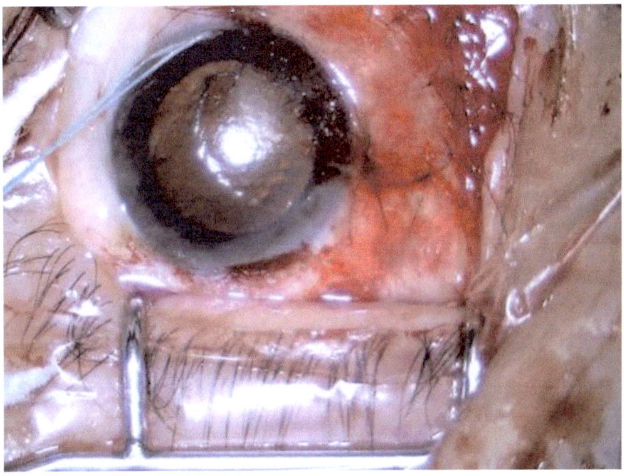

Fig. 7.21 Autologous conjunctival flap covers the surface of the fresh amniotic membrane, at which time the symblepharon is relieved, the lacrimal caruncle is reset, the scleral wound is covered with fresh amniotic membrane and conjunctival flap, and the corneal wound reaches 1/2 of the corneal area, which requires biological amniotic membrane covering

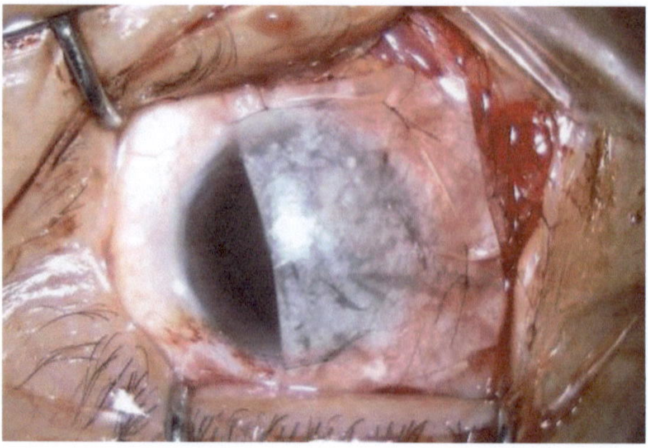

Fig. 7.22 Biological amniotic membrane covers the corneal and conjunctival wound

amnion may be partially sutured to the superior bulbar conjunctiva with 100 nylon suture.

9. Check: rinse the wounds with normal saline, and check for hematoma in the lacrimal caruncle area, good reattachment of lacrimal caruncle, active subconjunctival bleeding, smooth attachment of the transplanted conjunctiva to its graft bed, exposure of fresh bioamnion from the anastomosis, tight wrapping of corneal wounds by bioamnions, effusion and hematocele under bioamnions, and recovery of ocular mobility, etc. Gently squeeze the bulbar conjunctival graft and the corneal wound bioamnion with a medical sponge or cotton swab to remove the hematocele and effusion under the conjunctival flap and the bioamnion, enabling the conjunctival flap to tightly adhere to the sclera and the bioamnion to completely cover the corneal wound.

7.4 Part IV: Postoperative Management of Recurrent Pterygium

The postoperative management of the trilogy or tetralogy of recurrent pterygium is equivalent to that of basic and conventional pterygium operation, but special attention should be paid to the time of postoperative inflammation regression and the elimination of recurrent etiology:

1. Use of glucocorticoids: postoperative inflammation of recurrent pterygium usually lasts for a long time, requiring 6 weeks of glucocorticoids therapy, specifically with Tobramycin Dexamethasone Eye Drops (QID × 7d; TID × 7d; BID × 2w) for the first 4 weeks +0.1% Fluorometholone Eye Drops (BID × 2w) for the second 2 weeks; intraocular pressure changes should be monitored during treatment.
2. Treatment for acariasis and xerophthalmia: although there is no substantial data suggesting that recurrent pterygium is associated with demodicidosis, but

xerophthalmia and demodex blepharitis can exacerbate ocular surface inflammation. Therefore, strengthened treatment for demodicidosis and xerophthalmia is required after eliminating the recurrence associated with surgical methods, heredity, improper postoperative care and other factors.

3. Use of antimetabolites: antimetabolites may be administered temporarily for patients with recurrence following multiple excisions of pterygium, e.g., mitomycin C and 5FU; these drugs should be prescribed with caution or under the guidance of an experienced superior physician due to their high ocular surface toxicity. Patients should be followed up regularly during medication, and no use of antimetabolites is allowed if follow-up conditions are not met.

References

1. Fengming L, Lixin X. Chinese ophthalmology. 3rd ed. Beijing: People's Medical Publishing House; 2014. p. 1250–5.
2. Tejsu M, Jing J, Kai H. Clinical outcome of combined conjunctival autograft transplantation and amniotic membrane transplantation in pterygium surgery. Int J Ophthalmol. 2018;11(3):395400.
3. Jun S, Koichi K, Shigeto S, et al. Amniotic membrane transplantation with conjunctival autograft for recurrent pterygium. Ophthalmology. 2003;110(1):119124.

Chapter 8
Management of Surgical Complications Following Pterygium Surgery

Qingyan Zeng and Haoyu Wang

8.1 Section 1: Management of Intraoperative Events and Complications

8.1.1 Intraoperative Events and Management

8.1.1.1 Poor Exposure of the Surgical Field

The following are causes of a poor surgical field: inadequate adhesion of surgical drapes, poor patient coordination, narrow or abnormal palpebral fissures, inappropriate size of the eye speculum, symblepharon caused by recurrent pterygium, etc.

Prevention and resolution:

(a) Adhesive surgical drapes should be placed again to ensure even adherence to the eyelid skin and complete coverage of the eyelid margin.
(b) Traditional wire-type eyelid specula are usually unsuitable for eyes with extra-small palpebral fissures or abnormal eyelid morphology. Instead, an adjustable or Cook eyelid speculum should be used for eyelids varying in morphology to maximize surgical field exposure.
(c) In patients who cannot cooperate satisfactorily, a 5-0 nylon thread passing through the inferior corneal limbus can be used as a retraction suture to help fix the eyeball and fully expose the surgical field.
(d) In patients with symblepharon, the eye can be kept partially opened with an eyelid speculum or suture first, and after the adhesion is completely released, the eyelid speculum is fully opened to expose the surgical field.

Q. Zeng (✉) · H. Wang
Hankou Aier Eye Hospital, Wuhan, China

C. Wang, S. Li (eds.), *Pterygium Surgery*,
https://doi.org/10.1007/978-981-99-6843-5_8

8.1.1.2 Intraoperative Excessive Bleeding

Intraoperative bleeding is the most common complication of pterygium surgery due adjacent vascular tissue injury. Excessive bleeding can occur when the vascular tissue of the sheath of rectus muscles is damaged.

1. Preventive measures:

   (a) Blood pressure and blood sugar levels should be well controlled, and patients preoperative anxiety should be reduced.
   (b) In patients with a congestive and thick pterygium, local anti-inflammatory treatment (tobramycin-dexamethasone eye drops or 0.1% fluorometholone eye drops) should be given to effectively control inflammation prior to surgery.
   (c) A small amount of epinephrine can be added to anaesthetic drugs to enhance vascular contraction and reduce bleeding.
   (d) Large conjunctival vessels must be avoided during pterygium excision, and superficial scleral vessels should be avoided during suturing.
   (e) Pterygium tissue should be bluntly separated to avoid damage to the rectus muscles underneath.
   (f) Pterygium excision should be performed gently and properly to avoid damaging the adjacent caruncular tissue, which bleeds easily.

2. Treatment:

   (a) After identifying a bleeding site, compression or electrocoagulation is performed to stop the hemorrhage.
   (b) A pressure bandage is applied to the operated eye after the operation.

8.1.1.3 Issues Related to Superior Conjunctival Flap Grafting

1. The conjunctival flap is too large.

   An excessively large flap that exceeds the defect area after pterygium excision can wrinkle, affecting postoperative cosmetic outcomes and tear film coating.

   Prevention and resolution:

   Measure the bare scleral area using a ruler, and then, label the conjunctival area intended for flap use prior to harvesting. Match the sizes of the graft and the recipient bed by either trimming the conjunctival flap or enlarging the pterygium excision area.
2. The conjunctival flap is too small.

   When a flap is excessively small, i.e., smaller than the defect area after pterygium excision, excessively high suture tension easily causes tearing or separation of the flap, increasing the risk of pterygium recurrence.

   Preventive measures:

Measure the bare scleral area using a ruler, and then, label the conjunctival area intended to use for preparing a flap prior to harvesting. The bulbar conjunctiva is highly elastic; harvest the conjunctival flap without any fascial tissue and a size equal to or 0.25–0.5 mm smaller than the recipient bed.

Resolutions:

(a) In cases where the graft is slightly smaller than the defect area after pterygium excision, the surrounding conjunctiva may be stretched towards the cornea and fixed to the scleral tissue so that the bare scleral area is reduced to match the size of the graft.
(b) In cases where the graft is smaller than the defect area by 1.0 mm, another flap should be harvested from the superior conjunctiva and stitched together with the initial flap so that the total area matches the size of the defect area after pterygium excision. Alternatively, an amniotic membrane can be transplanted underneath and sutured together with the conjunctival graft to cover the bare scleral area.

3. The graft is brittle and cracks easily.

The conjunctiva is thin in elderly patients and patients with long-term chronic inflammation, and as a result, the harvested conjunctiva flap is brittle and easily cracks.

Preventive measures:

(a) In elderly patients, because the conjunctiva is thin, full-layer conjunctival tissue should be gently harvested and transferred with toothless microforceps or forceps that do not damage tissue to avoid graft rupture.
(b) The suture tension of the graft should be minimized to reduce the risk of cracking.
(c) Pterygium resection combined with biological amniotic membrane transplantation is recommended for elderly patients and patients with thin bulbar conjunctiva [1] (see Part IV of Chap. 6).

Resolutions:

If the graft has already cracked, amniotic membrane transplantation can be performed, or a biological amniotic membrane can be added to cover the scleral wound after flattening and placing the cracked conjunctival flap above the wound. The surgical procedures are described in Part IV of Chap. 6.

4. Confusing the sides of the conjunctival flap.

The two sides of the conjunctival flap may be difficult to distinguish during surgery due to poor exposure of the surgical field, excessive bleeding, operation errors, etc. If the fascial side of the grafted flap is facing upward, ischaemia and detachment of the graft are very likely to occur after surgery (Fig. 8.1).

Preventive measures:

(a) After being harvested, keep the conjunctival graft in the same position with the epithelial side facing upward and then slide it to the bare scleral area for suturing with the limbal margin facing towards the cornea.

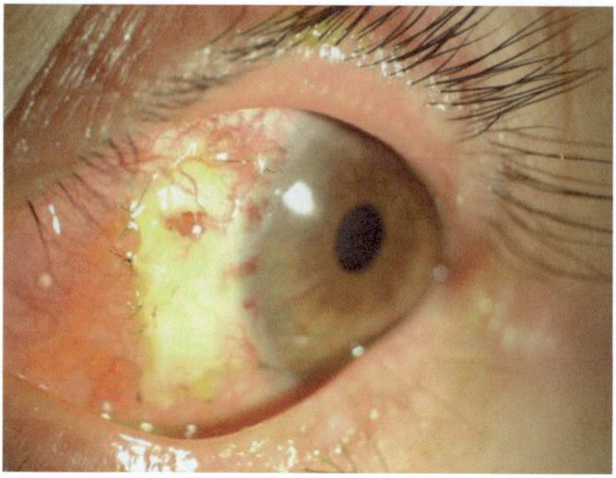

Fig. 8.1 Conjunctival implant fascia side up during implant inversion, at the fifth day after surgery, the implant is still ischemic and then falls off

(b) Identify the two sides of the graft microscopically at high magnification. The front side of the graft consists of smooth conjunctival epithelial tissue, and the back side contains some rough fascial tissue. In addition, use a moist cotton swab to swipe the graft surface for distinguishing sides: the smooth front side will not stick to the swab while the rough back side will.

Resolutions:

(a) In cases where incorrect upside-down placement of the graft is found at the early stage before epithelial growth, surgical treatment should be given as soon as possible. After the epithelial tissue that grows into the fascial surface of the graft and the surrounding bare scleral area is scraped off, the graft is reversed and sutured, with attention given to avoiding epithelial cyst formation during implantation.
(b) If the incorrect upside-down placement of the graft is found relatively in a delayed time, for example after 3 days, the conjunctival epithelium usually grows into the scleral surface under the graft, leading to an ischaemic state. In this case, treatments that control inflammation and facilitate wound repair should be administered; the sutures can be electively removed after the graft falls off on its own.

8.1.1.4 Difficulties in Making Sutures

Difficulties in making sutures during pterygium surgery may be caused by various factors, including poor patient cooperation, inadequate surgical field exposure, intraoperative bleeding, an excessively small graft size, and high brittleness of the graft.

Prevention and resolution:

(a) Patients who cannot cooperate due to nervousness can be administered tranquilizers or neuroleptic anaesthesia preoperatively and given oxygen inhalation to calm down the patient during surgery.
(b) Patients who cannot cooperate because of pain should be given a higher dose of anaesthetic agent. Alternatively, peribulbar/retrobulbar anaesthesia or even general anaesthesia can be used if necessary.
(c) For patients who cannot cooperate for other reasons, a retraction suture made at the lower limbus can be used to adjust the eye position for surgery.
(d) The handling of other issues can follow the descriptions in preceding sections.

8.1.1.5 Insufficient Clearing of the Corneal Wound Surface

For pterygium tightly adherent to the corneal surface or recurrent pterygium, the corneal wound after pterygium resection may retain some fibrous tissue; as a result, the corneal epithelium is difficult to repair, the tear film cannot be evenly coated, and the risk of infection and dry eyes becomes higher after surgery (Figs. 8.2 and 8.3).

Resolution: The fibrous tissue retained on the corneal surface is carefully removed with toothed microforceps, and the degenerated/opacified corneal area of recurrent pterygium can be properly scraped off with a fine circular blade to smoothen the corneal wound surface as much as possible without damaging the corneal stromal tissue. However, if the residual fibrous tissue is not in the pupillary area or the affected peripheral corneal tissue shows localized degeneration, overtreatment should be avoided. Instead, a thorough preoperative evaluation and full communication with the patient before surgery are necessary. The presence of residual fibrous tissue is more likely after surgical removal of pterygium with an infiltrative growth pattern.

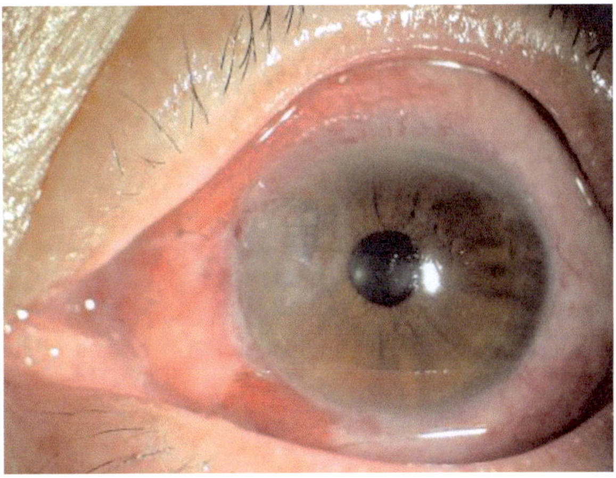

Fig. 8.2 Primary pterygium corneal surface treatment is not clean, and gray-white fibrous tissue residue is visible on the surface of the nasal corneal surface, which is uneven

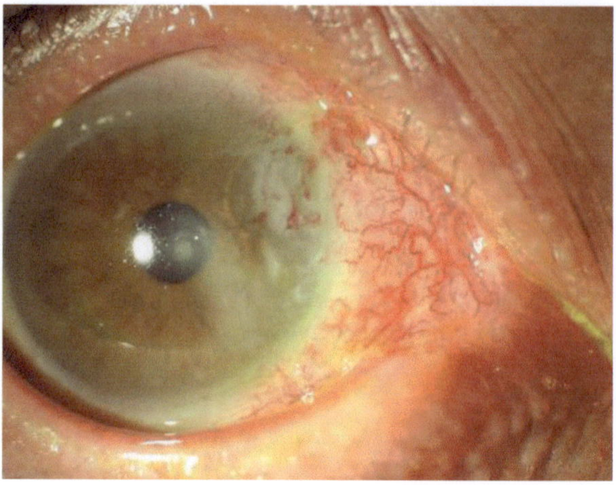

Fig. 8.3 Recurrent pterygium corneal surface treatment is not clean, and gray-white fibrous tissue residue is visible on the surface of the nasal corneal surface

8.1.2 Intraoperative Complications and Management

8.1.2.1 Complications Related to the Use of Anaesthetic Agents [2]

Local anaesthesia is the most common method used in pterygium surgery, and its complications mainly include systematic and ocular complications. Systemic complications include oculo-cardiac reflex responses, and ocular complications include subconjunctival hematoma, eyeball perforation, and rectus muscle injury.

Preventive measures:

(a) Oculo-cardiac reflex responses can be prevented to a certain extent by a gentle operation and avoidance of hypoxia and CO_2 accumulation.
(b) The injection of anaesthetic reagent should be performed by a specialist who is familiar with the anatomy of the eye under the patient's understanding and cooperation. The patient should be informed about slight pain before the injection to avoid sudden eye movements during the injection that might cause accidental injury to the eyeball. Attention should be given to avoiding conjunctival blood vessels when inserting needles. The needle should be advanced basically parallel to the eyeball wall. The operated eye should be in a horizontal and upward natural gaze position during injection. The slope side of the needle should face down, and the tip should be clearly visible below the conjunctiva.

Treatments [3]:

(a) When an ocular reflex response is present, surgery should temporarily halted, and the symptoms should be relieved or controlled by the intravenous injection of atropine.

(b) A small amount of subconjunctival hemorrhage can be stopped by compression without affecting the operation. For a large subconjunctival hematoma, the corresponding conjunctival area should be excised open to relieve the accumulated blood after bleeding is controlled by applying pressure.
(c) Perforation of the eyeball and injury of the rectus muscles are generally caused by operational errors. Injury severity should be assessed as soon as possible; an ocular fundus disease specialist should be consulted to assist in the treatment when eye penetration is suspected.

8.1.2.2 Conjunctival Tear

During pterygium surgery, tearing of the conjunctiva may occur due to an operation error or because the patient does not cooperate well and suddenly turns his or her eye.

Preventive measures and resolution:

For patients who cannot cooperate with satisfaction, a 5-0 nylon thread that passes through the inferior corneal limbus can be used as a retraction suture. The conjunctival tear can be aligned and sutured to restore the original anatomical structure.

8.1.2.3 Rectus Muscle Injury

Injury to the medial rectus muscle may occur during the injection of anaesthesia and excision of the pterygium body in pterygium surgery [4]. Injury to the medial rectus muscle, which attaches to the scleral tissue 5.5 mm from the limbus, can cause complications such as bleeding and diplopia.

Preventive measures:

Anaesthesia injection should be performed by a specialist who is familiar with the anatomy of the eye. After observing the eyeball position, the syringe needle should be advanced into the subconjunctival fibrovascular tissue. The needle tip should not be inserted too deep. For excision, the pterygium body and the sclera should be bluntly separated with attention to avoid damage to the sheath and body of the rectus muscle.

Treatments:

The rectus muscle injury should be treated with haemostasis and other symptomatic treatments, and the severed muscle must be sutured. Patients with severe injury may have eye movement disorders and diplopia after surgery. They should be proactively given anti-inflammatory medication and nutrition support. Surgical exploration and rectus muscle repair surgery should be performed if the symptoms remain after 3–6 months.

8.1.2.4 Corneal and Scleral Injuries

The cornea and the sclera might be damaged during separation of the pterygium head and body, respectively. In particular, damage is more likely in surgery for recurrent pterygium or pseudopterygium, which often have tissue adhesion and cause difficulties in identifying anatomic structures.

Preventive measures:

(a) The surgeon must be familiar with ocular anatomy. The head of a primary pterygium should be bluntly separated. During separation at the sclera, the blades of the scissors should be kept at a certain distance from the sclera and the rectus sheath above. Separation and resection must be performed under a clear view of the surgical field and anatomical structure.
(b) Before surgery for recurrent pterygium, the depth of the lesion should be carefully determined with a slit lamp and anterior segment OCT. Patients with a lesion exceeding 1/2 of the total thickness should be given lamellar keratoplasty. Over-separation should be avoided. Some scar tissue may remain on the cornea outside of the visual axis and the sclera to avoid corneal/scleral perforation caused by deep excision.
(c) For patients with atypical pterygium morphology, a detailed history of trauma and inflammation should be obtained before surgery. The cornea must be carefully examined under a slit lamp to rule out pseudopterygium caused by marginal corneal degeneration, Mooren's corneal ulceration, thermal burns, chemical injury, etc. During surgery, the corneal tissue should be managed cautiously and meticulously (Fig. 8.4).

Treatments:

(a) For patients with minor injuries, the involved eye can be packed with 0.3% ofloxacin ointment and a bandage soft contact lens and then covered with a pressure bandage.

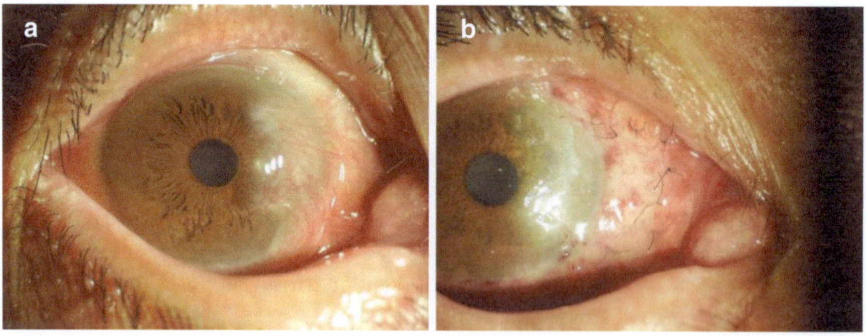

Fig. 8.4 Surgical outcomes of pseudopterygium. (**a**) Before surgery, a patient with a history of thermal burns had pterygium (wide head and irregular shape) growing into the cornea at 2 to 5 o'clock on the nasal side. (**b**) During surgery, the pseudopterygium tissue was carefully separated, followed by only limbal conjunctival flap autografting because the thickness of the cornea underneath was acceptable

(b) The corneal/scleral tissue that is lacerated or accidentally defective should be immediately aligned and sutured or treated with amniotic membrane stuffing/transplantation; if necessary, corneal/scleral transplantation and repair should be performed.
(c) For recurrent pterygium or pseudopterygium, amniotic membrane transplantation and lamellar keratoplasty are usually required for patients with a corneal wound depth greater than 1/3 and 1/2 CT after pterygium resection, respectively.

8.2 Section 2: Management of Postoperative Complications

8.2.1 Management of Early Postoperative Complications

8.2.1.1 Rupture of the Conjunctiva at the Anastomosis Site

Postoperative separation of the conjunctival graft, which often occurs at the nasal conjunctiva adjacent to the lacrimal caruncle, is caused by high tension and is mostly seen in young patients or patients with a thick pterygium (Figs. 8.5 and 8.6). It can also result from a loose limbal suture because the suture is not firmly secured.

Preventive measures:

(a) For patients with a congestive and thick pterygium, corticosteroid eye drops should be applied for 3–7 days to reduce inflammation before surgery. During surgery, the subconjunctival fascial tissue of the nasal side near the lacrimal caruncle should be fully excised, and the graft should be flattened, aligned and sutured with the nasal conjunctiva.
(b) The size of the graft should match the bare scleral area to avoid excessive suture tension. The graft should be secured with sutures that pass through the superficial layer of the sclera at four corners on the limbal and nasal sides.

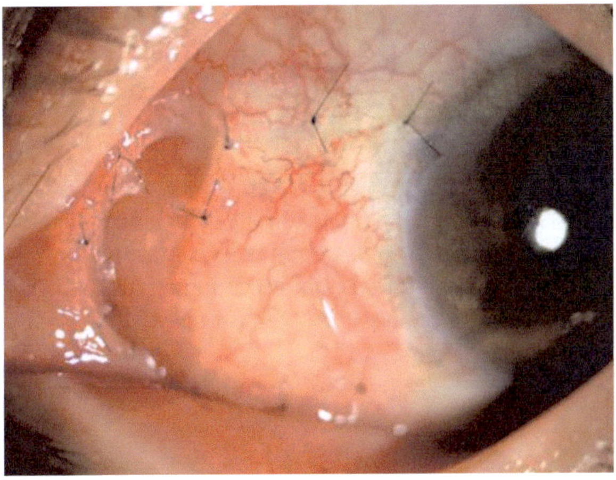

Fig. 8.5 Implant dehiscence at early postoperative period, and the dehiscence at the junction between the conjunctival implant and the conjunctiva at lacrimal caruncle at postoperative 1 week

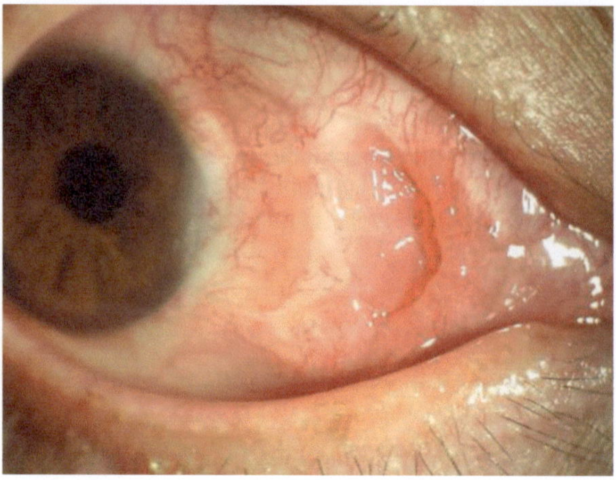

Fig. 8.6 Implant dehiscence, and the dehiscence at the junction between the conjunctival implant and the conjunctiva at lacrimal caruncle at postoperative 2 weeks, and the conjunctival epithelium grows into the dehiscence area

(c) The bulbar conjunctival tissues of the graft and recipient bed should be end-to-end anastomosed, avoiding the curling of the sutured edges.
(d) After surgery, patients, especially young patients, should avoid excessive eye movements, such as excessively turning the eye towards the temporal side.

Resolutions:

(a) A graft severely retreated due to loose sutures at the limbus should be re-sutured and returned to its proper position in a timely manner; otherwise, corneal epithelial repair will be affected, and the risk of recurrence will arise.
(b) Graft detachment occurs near the lacrimal caruncle at the nasal side mostly around the time of suture removal 7 days after surgery. Surgical treatment is unnecessary for a separated graft that has not detached. Eye drops and antibiotic eye ointment should be applied to promote epithelial repair so that the conjunctival area can epithelialize as soon as possible. Anti-inflammatory treatment (tobramycin-dexamethasone eye ointment) should be administered to prevent granuloma formation.

8.2.1.2 Persistent Oedema of the Conjunctival Graft

Postoperative oedema of the graft is more common in young patients, patients with excessive intraoperative operations (especially scleral surface cauterization for haemostasis), patients with a conjunctival graft with thick and excessive fascial tissue, and patients with an extra-large conjunctival graft or a graft with a limited expansion capacity because it is fixed on three sides with sutures that pass through the sclera tissue (Fig. 8.7).

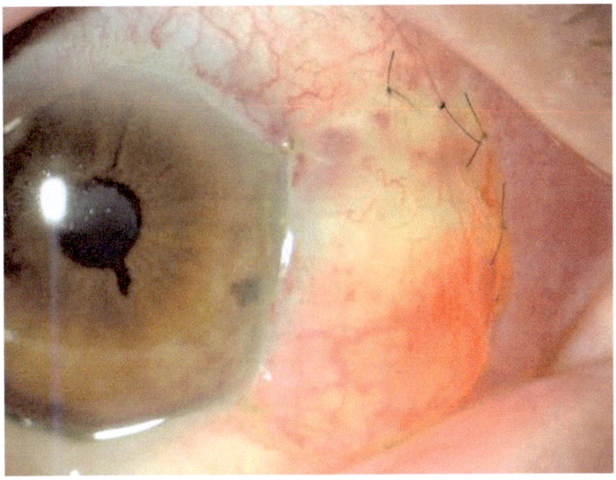

Fig. 8.7 Implant edema in a 45-year-old man who receives the surgery smoothly and shows implant edema at postoperative 3 days

Prevention measures:

The conjunctival flap should not include too much fascial tissue. Excessive cautery should be avoided during surgery; compression or low-dose epinephrine can be used as alternatives. The grafted conjunctival flap should not be too large and can be sutured to the recipient bed with the stitches passing through the superficial scleral tissue at four corners and stitches that do not pass through any scleral tissue for the remaining part.

Resolution:

Potent glucocorticoids and artificial tears can be applied appropriately, and attention should be given to changes in intraocular pressure.

8.2.1.3 Hematoma Underneath the Conjunctival Graft

Postoperative hematoma results from blood accumulation under the graft, which is common in patients who are elderly, have hypertension, receive excessive cauterization or epinephrine to stop bleeding during surgery, or hold their breath and cough forcefully after surgery (Fig. 8.8).

Prevention measures:

Excessive cautery should be avoided, and the use of epinephrine should be minimized during surgery. After surgery, attention should be given to stabilizing blood pressure, avoiding excessive movements, and avoiding excessive force and coughing.

Resolution:

A pressure bandage should be applied to the operated eye, and excessive eye movements should be avoided. Generally, haematomas are absorbed and subside without treatment in 3–7 days. Haemostatic drugs can be considered if necessary.

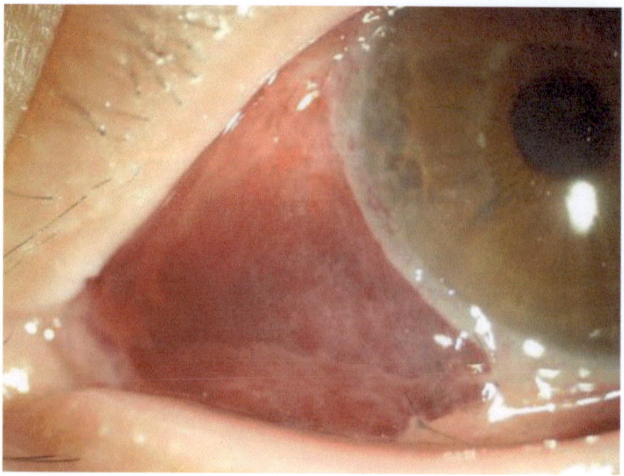

Fig. 8.8 Implant hematoma, the patient develops sudden hematoma under implant and coughs on the third day of postoperative

8.2.1.4 Persistent Corneal Epithelial Defects

Postoperative persistent corneal epithelial defects are present mostly in patients with severe dry eye, corneal dystrophy, limbal stem cell dysfunction, history of viral keratitis, diabetes, and abnormal eyelid morphologies (e.g., entropion/trichiasis and incomplete eyelid closure). They can also be caused by poor limbal conjunctival alignment of the graft during surgery.

Preventive measures:

(a) Conditions including eyelid abnormalities, severe dry eye, and limbal stem cell decompensation should be ruled out before pterygium surgery, which should not be performed until these conditions are managed properly.
(b) The conjunctival edge of the graft must be aligned well and sutured to the limbus during surgery (Fig. 8.9).
(c) The operated eye should be packed with antibiotic eye ointment (0.3% ofloxacin), high-quality preservative-free artificial tears (0.3% sodium hyaluronate), and eye fluid/gel containing growth factors after surgery for patients with rheumatoid disease, diabetes, thyroid disease, corneal dystrophy, herpes simplex virus keratitis, and dry eye. After the corneal epithelium is completely repaired, corticosteroids should be administered while closely monitoring the intraocular pressure and stability of the epithelium. For patients with a history of herpes simplex virus keratitis, antiviral drugs can be applied systemically or locally during the perioperative period to prevent the recurrence of viral infection.

Treatments:

(a) Generally, the corneal epithelium should be repaired 3 days after surgery; the causes for delayed repair must be identified and aggressively treated. Patients who have unrepaired corneal epithelial defects 1 week after surgery should be kept in the hospital for further monitoring.

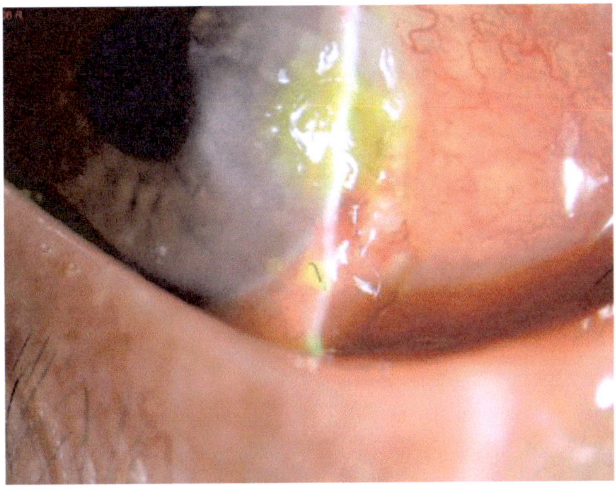

Fig. 8.9 Delayed healing of the corneal epithelium, the nasal corneal epithelium at 2 mm × 2 mm is still uncured on postoperative 6 days, the suture near the corneal limbus below the conjunctival implant is loose, and there is a significant gap between the implant and the corneal limbus

(b) Etiological treatments include drugs for dry eyes, antiviral drugs, immunosuppressants, etc. Eyelid abnormalities such as entropion and incomplete eyelid closure should be surgically treated. For cases in which the limbal conjunctival edge of the graft is not well aligned, a pressure bandage should first be applied over the affected eye; however, surgical realignment and suture must be performed in a timely manner if epithelial repair is unsatisfactory.

(c) The application of corticosteroids eye drops should be discontinued, and the involved eye should be packed with antibiotic eye ointment (0.3% ofloxacin) and deproteinized calf blood extract eye drops/gel; for severe cases, 20–50% autologous serum should be applied once an hour. The involved eye should be covered by a corneal bandage soft contact lens.

(d) If the corneal epithelial defect remains unrepaired after all above mentioned measures, amniotic membrane covering is recommended. Temporary/permanent tarsorrhaphy should be considered for patients with severe immune-related dry eye, aqueous-deficiency dry eye, or eyelid abnormalities.

8.2.1.5 Corneal Depressions

In patients with serious postoperative oedema of the conjunctival graft and the resultant uneven coating of the tear film on the ocular surface, the corneal limbal stroma adjacent to the graft might form a depression due to dehydration. The epithelium at the depression usually remains intact and shows fluorescein accumulation in fluorescein staining (Fig. 8.10).

Prevention measures:

The intended conjunctival graft should not be too thick, and excessive cauterization for haemostasis should be avoided during surgery. Patients with obvious

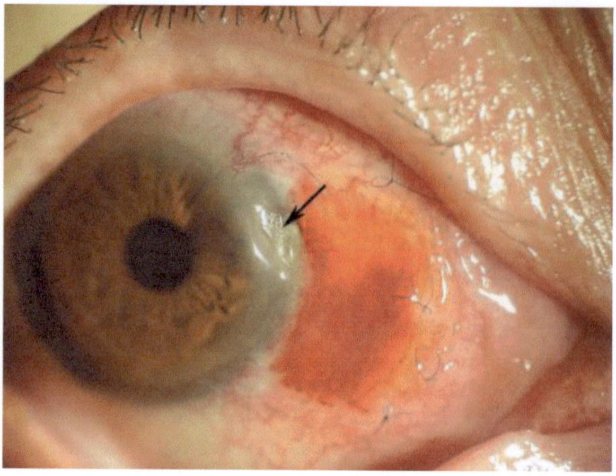

Fig. 8.10 Corneal. One week after surgery, there was a hematoma under the conjunctival graft, along with oedema of the graft. The adjacent limbal stroma formed a depression (black arrow) due to tissue dehydration

postoperative oedema of the graft should be treated with potent glucocorticoids to control inflammation. In addition, artificial tear gel can be applied four times a day, and the operated eye should be packed to avoid corneal dryness.

Resolution:

Corticosteroids should be discontinued when a significant corneal stromal depression occurs. The operated eye should be packed with preservative-free artificial tears and antibiotic eye ointment daily until the depressed site returns to its normal thickness.

8.2.1.6 Conjunctival Granuloma

Conjunctival granulomas are often caused by adverse events such as graft detachment and poor healing of the conjunctival surface, which induces local inflammation to stimulate proliferation of granulomatous tissue [5] (Fig. 8.11).

Prevention measures:

Special attention should be given to the harvesting and suturing of the graft to prevent the graft from detaching. If the graft is detached or the conjunctival epithelium does not heal, the involved eye should be packed with antibiotic eye ointment and artificial tear gel to promote rapid epithelial repair, and glucocorticoids should be properly applied to reduce inflammation.

Resolution:

Conjunctival granulomas can be removed from their base, followed by cauterization of the base. After surgery, potent corticosteroids and artificial tears should be applied until inflammation is controlled and the conjunctival epithelium is completely repaired.

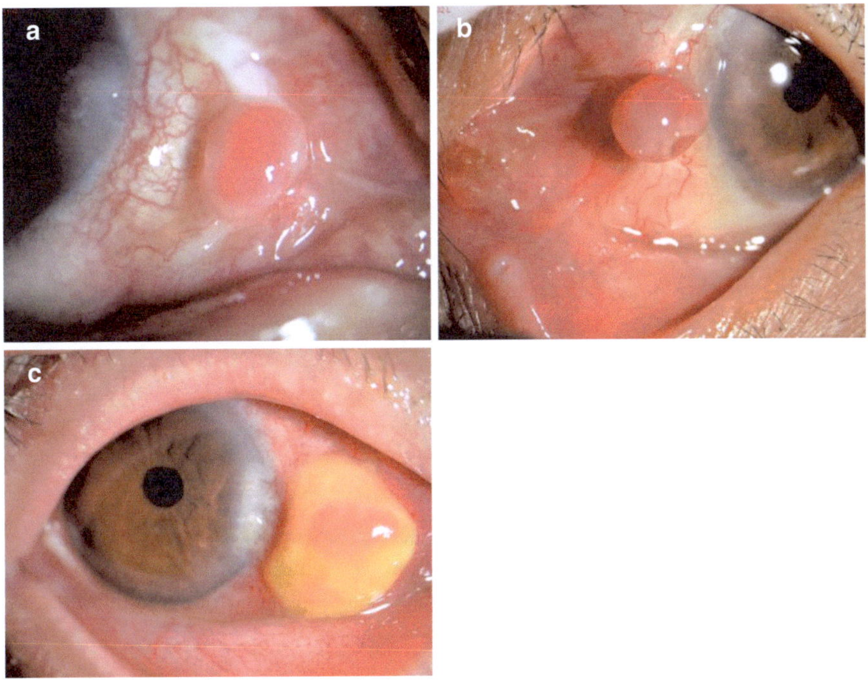

Fig. 8.11 Conjunctival granuloma. (**a**–**c**) Within 1–3 weeks after surgery, granulomatous tissue grew at the nasal wound of the conjunctival graft. Graft detachment was visible in the early stage, and the surrounding subconjunctival tissue hyperplasia proliferated in the later stage

8.2.1.7 Foreign Body Sensation

Postoperative foreign body **sensation** is generally caused by excessive intraoperative bleeding, cotton fibres/threads or other foreign matter left due to an unclear surgical field or careless operation, and necrotic/degenerative tissue due to excessive cauterization. Foreign body **sensation** can cause a postoperative inflammatory response (Fig. 8.12).

Prevention measures:

(a) The operation should be performed gently to avoid excessive tissue damage and severe bleeding during surgery.
(b) Cautery for haemostasis should be avoided as much as possible, and necrotic tissue must be removed.
(c) Haemostatic materials such as cotton pads should not be too small, and their edges should be trimmed to avoid the fall-off of loose cotton fibres.
(d) After surgery, the surgical field should be carefully inspected to remove foreign material, such as residual cotton fibres and threads.

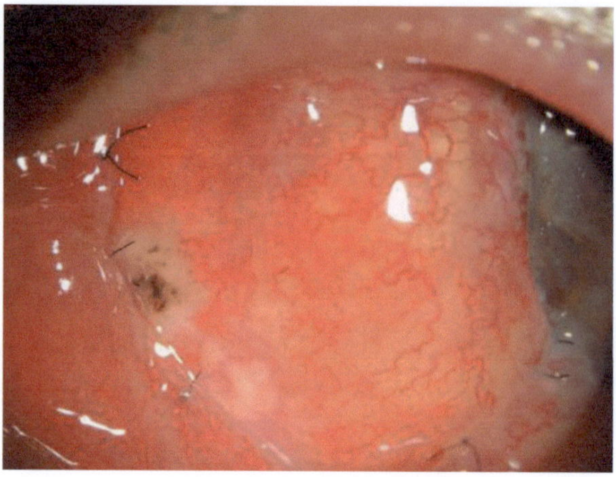

Fig. 8.12 Necrotic residue, excessive intraoperative cauterization to stop bleeding, causing necrotic residue and forming inflammatory reaction at surrounding tissue

Resolution:

Foreign material (e.g., cotton fibres) left after surgery should be carefully removed to avoid secondary damage; if there is an inflammatory response, anti-inflammatory drugs can be added for symptomatic and supportive treatment.

8.2.1.8 Corneal and Scleral Dissolution

Corneal dissolution occurs mostly in patients with (1) persistent corneal epithelial defects caused by various reasons that are not treated in time; (2) long-term excessive use of glucocorticoids; (3) severe dry eyes before surgery, especially immune-related dry eyes, which often lead to corneal perforation in severe cases; and (4) diabetes.

Scleral dissolution [6] occurs mostly in patients who undergo excessive cauterization to stop bleeding and use antimetabolites such as mitomycin and 5-fluorouracil [7] (Figs. 8.13 and 8.14).

Prevention measures:

Scleral cautery for haemostasis should be avoided as much as possible during surgery, and the use of antimetabolic drugs should be avoided. Generally, the corneal epithelium can be repaired 3 days after surgery; the causes for delayed repair must be identified and aggressively treated until full healing of the corneal epithelium. Unrepaired conjunctival epithelial defects and the bare scleral area should also be treated as soon as possible until the conjunctival epithelium is repaired.

Resolutions [8]:

(a) Once corneal and scleral dissolution is diagnosed, the first step should be to rule out fungal, bacterial, and other pathogen infections by confocal microscopy of fungal and bacterial cultures from scraped tissue.
(b) The causes of corneal and scleral dissolution must be identified and treated; for example, antiviral drugs should be given to treat dry eyes, and herpetic stromal

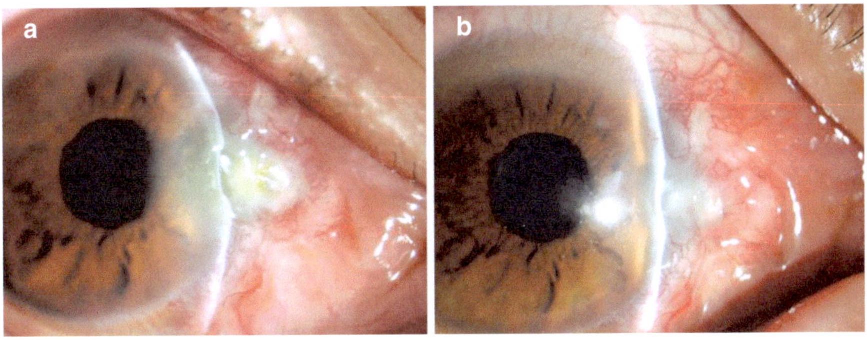

Fig. 8.13 Postoperative corneal and scleral dissolution. (**a**) Three weeks after surgery, a patient with diabetes presented dissolution of the cornea and adjacent scleral tissue to the deep stromal layer. (**b**) Use of glucocorticoids was discontinued in favour of 0.3% ofloxacin eye ointment and 0.3% sodium hyaluronate eye drops, which were applied to the involved eye 4 times per day. After 5 days of treatment, corneal and scleral dissolution was alleviated, and the stroma remained significantly depressed and thinned

Fig. 8.14 Corneal dissolution. In the rheumatoid patient at 1 month after pterygium surgery, the central cornea below the nose is dissolved and perforated, with iris incarceration and anterior chamber obliteration

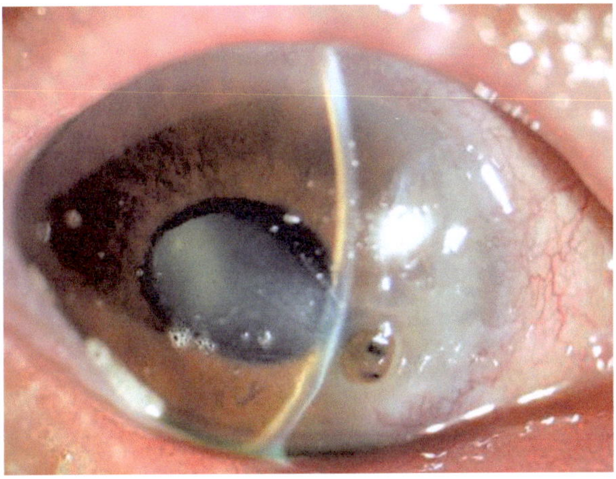

keratitis (HSK) and immunosuppressants should be given to treat rheumatic and other diseases of the immune system.

(c) Use of corticosteroids should be discontinued immediately, and the involved eye should be packed with antibiotic eye ointment and high-quality artificial tears. Noninfectious keratopathy and near-limbal scleral lesions can be treated with a bandage soft contact lens.

(d) Severe corneal dissolution can be treated with amniotic membrane covering or even conjunctival flap covering. Severe scleral dissolution should be treated with scleral repair surgery, and the transplanted scleral graft should be covered with a conjunctival flap to avoid scleral graft ischaemia and second dissolution.

(e) Patients with corneal perforation should undergo fibrin glue-assisted multilayer amniotic membrane transplantation in a timely manner, which can be combined with lamellar keratoplasty for patients with large stromal defects (Fig. 8.15). Penetrating keratoplasty should be avoided as much as possible because it may cause a series of complications, such as corneal graft dissolution and rejection.

8.2.1.9 Dry Eye

The causes for dry eye early after surgery [9] mostly include the following:

1. Excision of a large area of conjunctival tissue during pterygium surgery, causing a decrease in the number of goblet cells [10] and mucin secretion;
2. Improper intraoperative operation or excessive operation time, resulting in dryness and damage to the ocular surface;

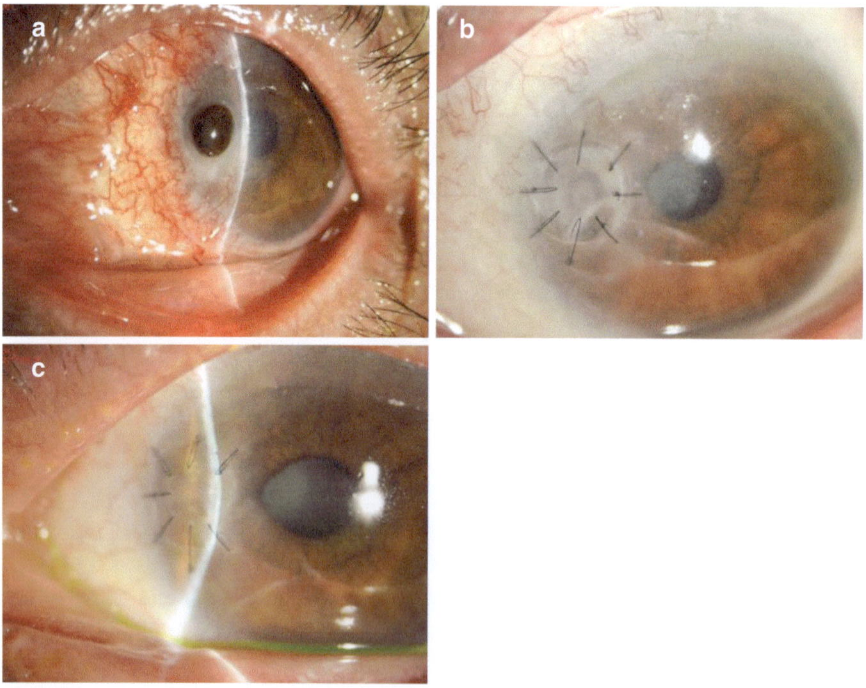

Fig. 8.15 Corneal dissolution and perforation after pterygium surgery. (**a**) In the rheumatoid patient at 3 weeks after pterygium surgery, conjunctival implant heals well, nasal peripheral cornea dissolves and perforates, with iris incarceration and nasal anterior chamber obliteration; (**b**) interlaminar amniotic membrane transplantation combined with laminar keratoplasty are performed. At postoperative 1 week, the implant has mild edema, good alignment, with no double anterior chambers and with basically round pupil; (**c**) at postoperative 10 months, corneal implant becomes transparent, and anterior chamber is well formed, without anterior synechiae of iris

3. Postoperative tissue oedema and uneven ocular surface, resulting in uneven coating and thereby low stability of the tear film;
4. Postoperative inflammatory responses and the use of drugs such as corticosteroids and antibiotics, further damaging the ocular surface; and
5. MGD prior to pterygium surgery.

Prevention measures:

The size of the excised area and the conjunctival flap should be reasonable, and the operation should be gentle to avoid damaging healthy ocular surface tissue. During surgery, moist cotton pads should be used to cover the non-operated corneal and conjunctival areas to protect the ocular surface. After surgery, medication should be given reasonably, and drugs with low toxicity to the ocular surface should be used as much as possible.

Resolution:

Anti-inflammatory treatment should be applied appropriately to reduce ocular surface reactions such as inflammation and oedema, with avoidance of the prolonged use of glucocorticoids. Preservative-free artificial tears/gel should be applied four times per day, and drugs (e.g., diquafosol sodium eye drops) that promote mucin secretion should be applied six times per day.

8.2.1.10 Infections

1. Bacterial infection [11]:

   Postoperative bacterial infection of the operated eye occurs mostly in patients with poor eye hygiene who have chronic ocular surface inflammation, such as trachoma, blepharitis, and chronic dacryocystitis, before surgery. Other risk factors include persistent corneal epithelial defects, trauma, severe dry eye, and diabetes after surgery (Fig. 8.16).

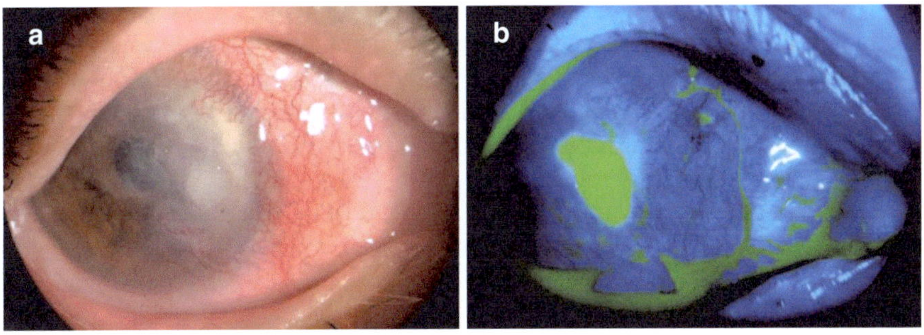

Fig. 8.16 Bacterial corneal ulceration after pterygium surgery. (**a**) One month after surgery, a patient with diabetes had eye redness and pain for 2 weeks. The conjunctival graft remained in place and was flat, and the superonasal peripheral cornea was degenerated. A corneal ulcer with stromal infiltration was visible at 3 o'clock near the limbus and was later confirmed as G+ coccus infection by tissue scraping examination. (**b**) Positive fluorescein staining

Preventive measures:

Ocular surface abnormalities, such as trachoma, dacryocystitis, and blepharitis, should be aggressively treated with antibiotics and physical cleaning prior to surgery. In patients with dacryocystitis, pterygium surgery should be postponed until the inflammation is completely controlled after lacrimal surgery. Patients with persistent corneal epithelial defects after surgery should be hospitalized for observation until the epithelium is completely repaired.

Resolutions:

(a) Pathogens must be identified as much as possible by confocal microscopy of cultures from scraped tissue.
(b) The use of corticosteroids should be discontinued, and antibacterial treatment should be aggressively applied based on the results of tissue scraping examination. For cases in which laboratory evidence for bacterial infection is insufficient and other pathogens, such as fungi, have been ruled out, empirical diagnosis-driven therapy can be considered. If treatment is not effective, medication should be adjusted based on the results of drug sensitivity testing.
(c) Patients for whom the severe infection involves the cornea and sclera and cannot be effectively controlled with medication should undergo conjunctival flap covering in a timely manner.
(d) For cases in which the infection is effectively controlled but ulcer healing is delayed, autologous serum can be added into the treatment regimen, as can amniotic membrane covering if necessary (Fig. 8.17).

2. Fungal infection [12]:

   The risk factors for fungal infection include poor eye hygiene, postoperative corneal conjunctival epithelial defects, trauma, and diabetes, as well as prolonged topical application of glucocorticoids and wearing of a bandage soft contact lens (Fig. 8.18).

   Preventive measures:

   After surgery, patients should be educated to maintain good hygiene of the involved eye and prevent trauma or contamination through dirty water. Patients with persistent corneal epithelial defects should be hospitalized for observation until the epithelium is completely repaired. The bandage soft contact lens should be removed after healing of the corneal epithelium and should not stay in the eye for too long. Corticosteroids should not be used for too long, generally for approximately 1 month after surgery, and the dose should gradually be reduced on the basis of the inflammation status of the eye. Patients with diabetes, severe dry eyes, etc., should be followed up regularly once per week for a month.

   Resolution:

   The use of corticosteroids should be discontinued immediately. Pathogens must be identified as much as possible by culturing tissue specimens scraped from lesions and examining the cultures under a confocal microscope; based on the results, the patient is given aggressive antifungal therapy, generally 5% nata-

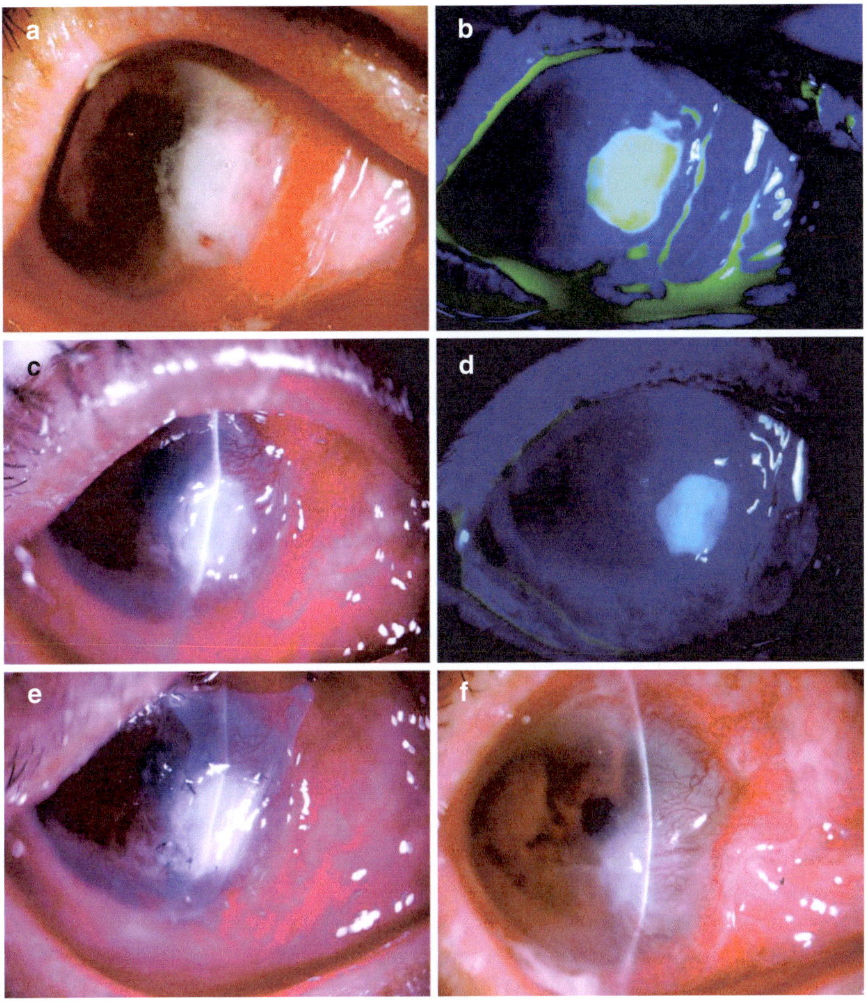

Fig. 8.17 Bacterial infection after pterygium surgery. (**a**, **b**) One month after pterygium surgery, a patient had eye redness and pain for half of a month. The narrow and long nasal conjunctival graft remained in place. There was visible degeneration and infiltration of the nasal corneal stroma, accompanied by a 3 mm × 5 mm ulcer covered with yellow–white necrotic tissue. G+ cocci were detected in the tissue specimen scraped from the ulcer. (**c**, **d**) Gatifloxacin eye drops and tobramycin eye drops were given alternately; after 6 days of treatment, although the ulcer lesion had a cleaner surface and shrunk slightly, improvement was slow. The bacterial culture results suggested *Micrococcus luteus* infection. (**e**) The patient underwent debridement of ulcer foci combined with amniotic membrane covering. The amniotic membrane remained in place 1 day after surgery. (**f**) Two weeks after amniotic membrane covering, the amniotic membrane was removed. The corneal ulcer had healed, the cornea showed remarkable neovascularization, and the stroma had mild opacity and oedema. The proliferation of the nasal conjunctival tissue affected the limbus

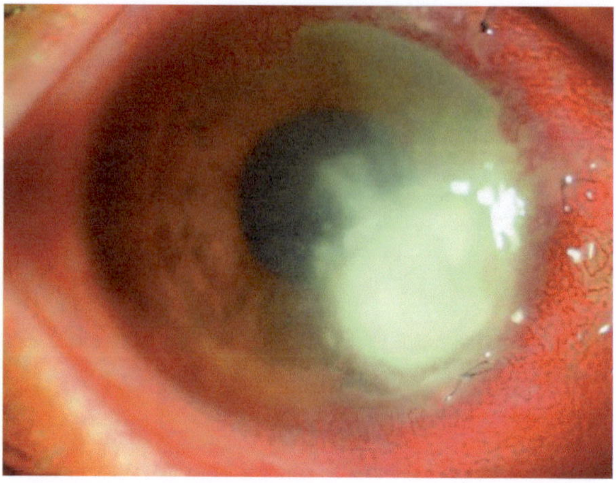

Fig. 8.18 Fungal infection after pterygium surgery. At 1 week after pterygium surgery, a large area of nasal corneal ulceration is observed, with cheese-like necrotic changes on the surface, clear boundaries, and a large number of fungal hyphae on scrapings

mycin eye drops and 1% voriconazole eye drops once per hour. If the infection cannot be controlled effectively by medication, debridement combined with conjunctival flap covering should be given in a timely manner (Fig. 8.19).

3. Recurrence of viral infection:

   For patients with preoperative corneal viral infections, factors including surgical stimulation and glucocorticoid application may activate viruses and lead to the recurrence of inflammation.

   Preventive measures:

   Before surgery, a detailed medical history and information regarding whether there is a history of repeated episodes of eye redness and pain should be obtained. The patients should be carefully examined under a slit lamp for corneal abnormalities such as corneal nebula, macula, and neovascularization (Figs. 8.20 and 8.21).

   For some patients, the corneal lesion may be located below the pterygium, and inflammation stimulates pterygium growth, often leading to irregular morphology and pseudopterygium (Fig. 3.37). For patients who have a history of the abovementioned signs and symptoms, the possibility of viral keratitis should be highly suspected, for which topical antiviral drugs should be applied after surgery until the use of corticosteroids, eye drops is discontinued; oral antiviral drugs should be given to patients who had severe episodes previously. The patients should be followed up closely, generally once per week in the first month after surgery.

   Treatments:

   Both systemic and topical antiviral therapy should be given once the recurrence of viral infection is suspected. Corticosteroids can be applied if necessary. High-quality artificial tears and neurotrophic drugs (e.g., vitamin B1 and vitamin B12) can also be used. Immunosuppressants such as tacrolimus/cyclosporine eye drops can be added to the treatment regimen if viral infection causes stromal necrosis or affects the epithelium.

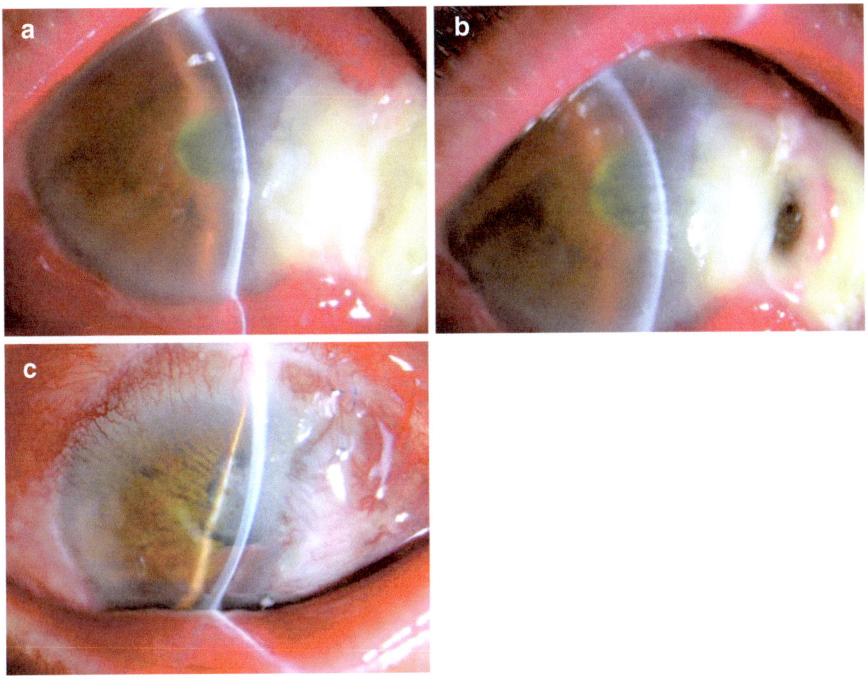

Fig. 8.19 Corneal and scleral fungal infection after pterygium surgery. (**a**) A 65-year-old patient from a rural area had only one seeing eye. One month after pterygium, the patient reported a history of injury by vegetative matter and eye redness and pain for 1 week. The patient's visual acuity was HM. There was a 6 mm × 3 mm grey–white ulcerous lesion in the nasal cornea and a 6 mm × 5 mm ulcerous lesion on the nasal sclera, which were covered by a large amount of yellow–white necrotic matter. The anterior chamber was moderately deep and contained grey–white exudates. There were adhesions behind the pupil, and the lens was opaque. The tissue specimen scraped from the ulcerous lesion contained only a large number of neutrophils. (**b**) After 3 days of intensive antibacterial therapy, the patient had limbal perforation, iris incarceration, worsened corneal oedema, and deteriorated anterior chamber inflammation. Fungal culture indicated *Fusarium* spp. (**c**) Conjunctival flap covering combined with two anterior chamber injections of liposomal amphotericin B. Half a month after the second injection, the patient could count fingers at 10 cm, the nasal conjunctival flap remained in place, with sufficient blood flow, the central cornea was transparent, there was no obvious inflammatory response in the anterior chamber, and post-iris tissue adhesions were present in the pupillary area

8.2.1.11 Conjunctival Cysts

The most common type of conjunctival cysts is implantation cysts that form due to the implantation of corneal epithelium underneath a conjunctival graft (Fig. 8.22).

Prevention measures:

After pterygium excision, the corneal wound and bare scleral area should be thoroughly rinsed to avoid the retention of epithelial tissue or foreign bodies under the conjunctival graft.

Resolution:

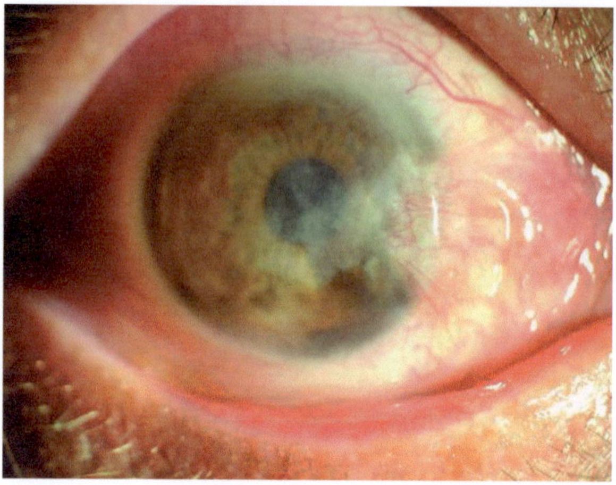

Fig. 8.20 Pterygium with macula cornea. The patient has a history of recurrent eye redness and pain, highly suspected viral keratitis. Ganciclovir eye drops solution is given after pterygium surgery, and no recurrence of keratopathy is observed during follow-up period

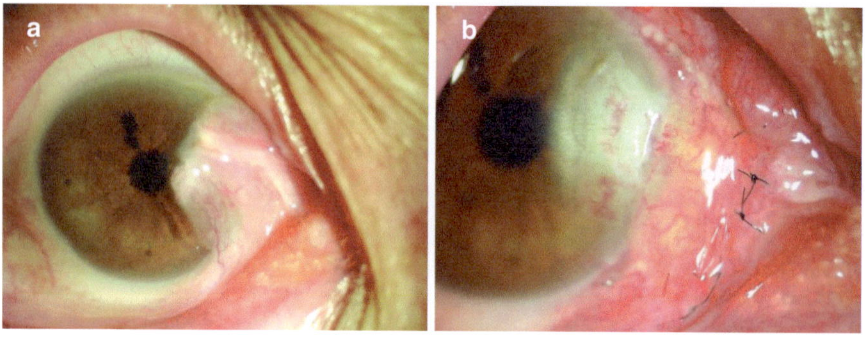

Fig. 8.21 Stromal keratitis accompanied by pseudopterygium. (**a**) The hypertrophic and proliferative nasal conjunctiva grew into the cornea, forming a pseudopterygium with a wide head extending above the nose. The patient had a history of repeated "eye inflammation". (**b**) After surgery, the superior nasal corneal stroma was opaque and neovascularized, and the near-limbus area was infiltrated. The patient was given acyclovir tablets orally combined with ganciclovir eye drops, and corticosteroids were added after epithelial healing. The patient's condition was stable during the follow-up period

Small cysts can be treated with puncture and potent anti-inflammatory treatment. Corticosteroids and nonsteroidal anti-inflammatory eye drops can be used for 1–2 weeks to reduce the risk of recurrence. Large cysts or recurrent cysts after cyst puncture has already been performed can be surgically removed while separating and preserving healthy conjunctival tissue as much as possible.

8.2.1.12 Acute Angle-Closure Glaucoma Attack

For patients with shallow anterior chamber or chronic angle-closure glaucoma, an acute glaucoma attack may be triggered by factors such as surgical stimulation, the intraoperative application of epinephrine for pupil dilation, and postoperative eye

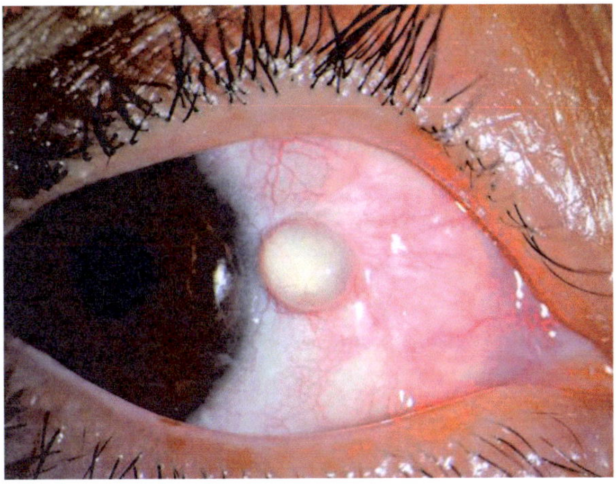

Fig. 8.22 Conjunctival cyst. At 1 month after pterygium surgery, hyaline cystic mass is visible under the conjunctival implant

packing. Glaucoma attacks occur more frequently during the early postoperative period or even the night of surgery.

Prevention measures:

(a) Prevention should be the mainstay. The peripheral depth of the anterior chamber and intraocular pressure should be examined before surgery. In cases in which the peripheral anterior chamber depth is less than 1/3 CT, ultrasound biomicroscopy (UBM) and gonioscopy should be performed, and a glaucoma specialist should be consulted. Laser iridotomy should be performed or a pupil-constricting drug should be applied to the involved eye during the perioperative period to prevent an acute glaucoma attack if necessary.
(b) For patients with a shallow anterior chamber, the conjunctival graft should be harvested from the inferior area as much as possible to keep the superior conjunctiva intact for future antiglaucoma surgery, such as trabeculectomy.
(c) For patients with a shallow anterior chamber, the use of epinephrine should be avoided during surgery to avoid pupil dilation that might induce glaucoma.

Resolution:

For patients who are undergoing an acute glaucoma attack, both systematic and topical treatments should be given to lower intraocular pressure and induce pupil constriction; additionally, attention should be given to monitoring the contralateral eye and preventing attacks in both eyes.

8.2.2 Management of Long-Term Postoperative Complications

8.2.2.1 Pterygium Recurrence

There is a possibility of recurrence after any type of pterygium surgery. Risk factors [13] include age less than 40 years, being female, second surgery after recurrence, pterygium congestion, thick pterygium, dry eyes, *Demodex* blepharitis, severe postoperative conjunctival reaction, dust in the postoperative living environment, and ultraviolet stimulation, etc.

Generally, the recurrence rate is 2–5% for pterygium resection combined with autologous limbal stem cell transplantation, 10–37.5% for pterygium resection combined with amniotic membrane transplantation, and as high as 20–70% for simple resection (Figs. 8.23 and 8.24).

Preventive measures:

(a) To avoid long-term recurrence after surgery, attention should be given to avoiding risk factors before and during surgery, including proper preoperative medication to keep pterygium quiescent and the careful and complete removal of pterygium tissue during surgery.

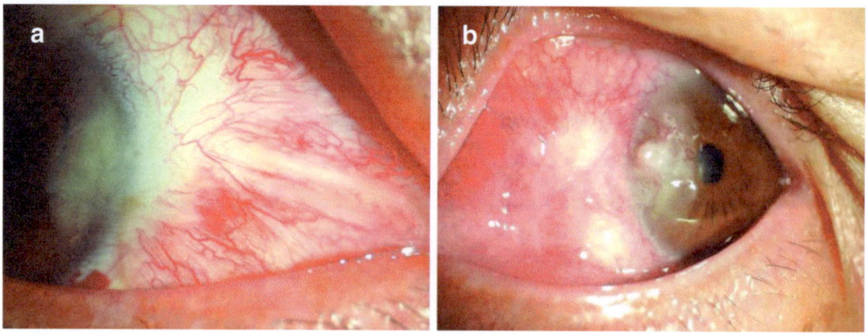

Fig. 8.23 Pterygium recurrence (tendency) after surgery. (**a**) Two months after amniotic membrane transplantation, the membrane tissue was generally absorbed, and the nasal subconjunctival fibrovascular tissue was hyperplastic and grew towards the limbus, indicating pterygium recurrence. (**b**) More than 2 months after amniotic membrane transplantation, the nasal amniotic membrane remained visible, and a portion of fibrovascular tissue grew into the cornea fibrovascular membranes to form an obvious bulge, indicating recurrent pterygium

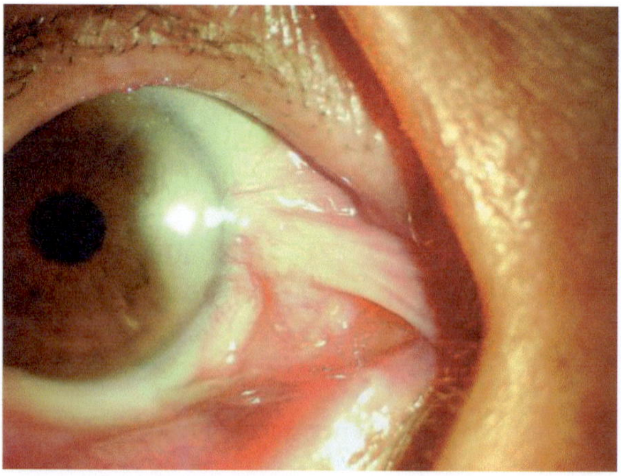

Fig. 8.24 Recurrence after pterygium surgery. At 6 months after simple pterygium excision, the fibrovascular tissue below the nasal conjunctiva is hypertrophied, the head has reached the corneal limbus, and the lacrimal caruncle is displaced towards the corneal limbus

(b) After surgery, anti-inflammatory drugs should be appropriately used on the basis of the patient's condition. For young patients, patients with thick pterygium, and patients with chronic inflammation of the ocular surface, tobramycin-dexamethasone eye drops should be applied for 1 month, followed by 0.1% fluorometholone eye drops for 2 weeks; attention should be given to changes in intraocular pressure.
(c) Patients should avoid strong ultraviolet radiation, wind, sand, tobacco, alcohol, and spicy food within 3–6 months after surgery.
(d) Pterygium recurrence occurs mostly within 1 year after surgery; therefore, follow-up should last at least 1 year.

Resolutions:

(a) Patients showing early pterygium recurrence can be given stronger anti-inflammatory treatment (Fig. 8.25). The use of corticosteroids can be extended to 3 months or later postoperatively and can be replaced with nonsteroidal anti-inflammatory drugs along with close follow-up if the patient's intraocular pressure is high.
(b) Drugs suppressing vascular endothelial growth factor can be injected subconjunctivally to reduce neovascularization.
(c) For patients with pterygium recurrence, a second surgery can be considered 6–12 months after the initial surgery but should not occur earlier than 6 months postoperatively, especially for patients who have had recurrence multiple times.
(d) Generally, surgical resection of recurrent pterygium should be combined with autologous limbal conjunctival transplantation (Fig. 8.26). For patients

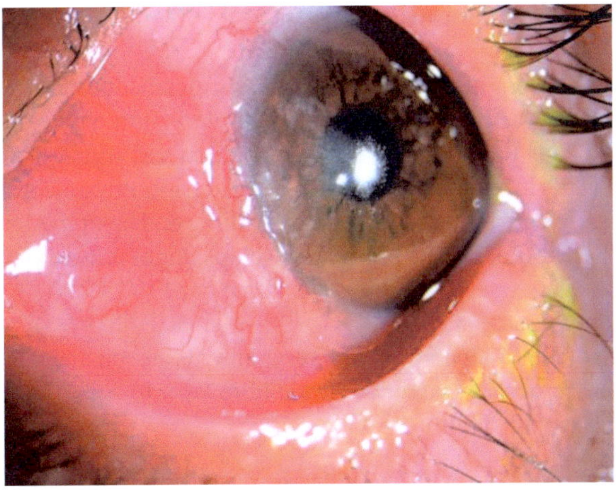

Fig. 8.25 Recurrence tendency. At 3 months after pterygium excision combined with conjunctival limbal autograft transplantation, the conjunctival implant is small and significantly constricted; the fibrovascular tissue below the nasal conjunctiva is hypertrophied and grows towards corneal limbus. It is recommended to strength anti-inflammatory therapy to prevent the recurrence of the pterygium

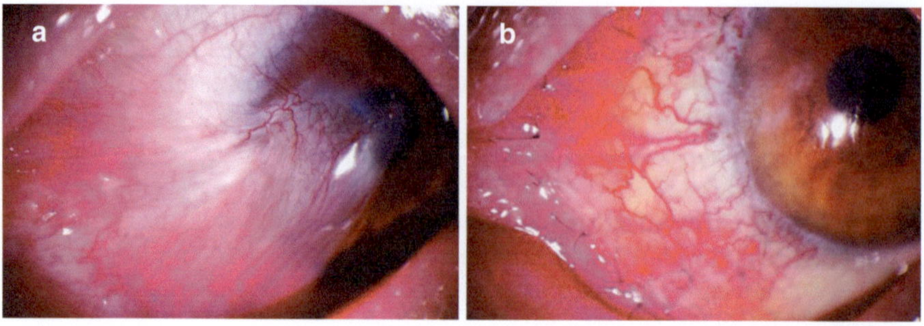

Fig. 8.26 Before and after surgery for recurrent pterygium. (**a**) A patient with recurrent pterygium had conjunctival scarring, along with abundant subconjunctival fibrovascular tissue, which invaded the cornea approximately 4 mm. (**b**) One week after recurrent pterygium resection combined with limbal conjunctival flap autograft, the conjunctival graft was flat and aligned well with the defect

who have had recurrence multiple times and do not have any healthy limbal tissue, surgical resection should be performed along with a conjunctival flap autograft, which can also be combined with amniotic membrane transplantation if the conjunctival defect is too large. Simple amniotic membrane transplantation is not suitable because of an extremely high probability of pterygium recurrence. The intraoperative use of mitomycin/5-fluorouracil can reduce the chance of recurrence, but there is a risk of postoperative scleral thinning and dissolution; therefore, mitomycin/5-fluorouracil should be used with caution.

8.2.2.2 Corneal Astigmatism

Patients with pterygium may develop corneal astigmatism due to various factors, including the pulling and compression effect of pterygium on the cornea, the lensing effect of the local tear film, and the degeneration and scarring of subpterygium corneal tissue [14]. In addition, the excessive excision of corneal tissue can also cause corneal astigmatism. After surgery, the pulling and compression of the cornea by pterygium is relieved, but the scar that develops might remain and cause corneal astigmatism.

Prevention measures:

Intraoperative blunt separation of pterygium tissue on the cornea generally should not break through the anterior elastic fibre layer to avoid the removal of corneal stromal tissue with a knife.

Resolution:

The patient should be monitored for more than 3 months, and eye drops/gel containing growth factors should be given to help with tissue repair. After 3 months, comprehensive optometry should be performed, and glasses should be prescribed if the astigmatism has stabilized; rigid gas permeable (RGP) lenses can be prescribed for severe irregular astigmatism.

8.2.2.3 Dry Eye

The common causes of postoperative long-term dry eye include uneven coating of the tear film on the ocular surface due to postoperative corneal and/or conjunctival scarring and the presence of preoperative dry eye.

Prevention measures:

(a) For patients with dry eye symptoms before surgery, a full set of dry eye examinations should be performed to assess severity. Pterygium surgery can be performed in patients with moderate dry eyes after dry eye symptoms and signs are controlled and stabilized. For severe dry eyes, pterygium surgery should be postponed until the cause is identified and properly managed.
(b) During surgery, it is critical to obtain a smooth corneal surface after removing the above pterygium tissue, and then evenly align the conjunctival graft and the conjunctiva of the recipient bed so that the ocular surface can return to a smooth appearance and the tear film can be coated evenly after surgery.

Resolution:

For patients with an unsmooth ocular surface, high-quality artificial tear gel can be given to relieve symptoms. For severe cases, the scar tissue can be surgically removed. Patients should undergo further examinations to identify the dry eye type for targeted treatment.

8.2.2.4 Late-Onset Infection

Prolonged high-dose corticosteroids may cause late-onset infections, especially fungal infections. The details of bacterial infections, fungal infections, and the recurrence of viral infections are discussed in Sect. 8.2 of this chapter.

Prevention measures:

Corticosteroids should not be used for too long. Generally, they should be used for approximately 1 month after surgery and then gradually reduced on the basis of the inflammatory status of the eye.

Resolution:

Tissue scraping, culture, and confocal microscopy should be performed to identify pathogens. The use of glucocorticoids should be discontinued immediately, and proper treatment should be provided based on test results.

8.2.2.5 Cosmetic Complaints

The reasons for patient complaints of cosmetic appearance include the following:

1. The cornea is not smooth due to residual tissue of the pterygium head;
2. The degenerative corneal tissue beneath the pterygium appears greyish white (mostly occurs in long-growing pterygia) (Figs. 8.27 and 8.28);

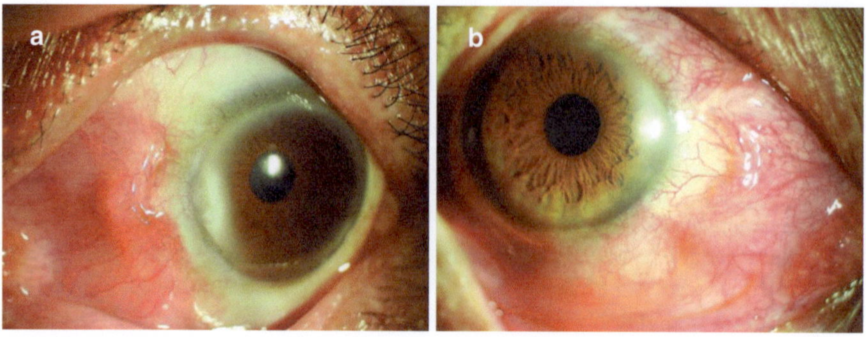

Fig. 8.27 An excessively small conjunctival graft. (**a**, **b**) Because the conjunctival graft was too small, the surrounding subconjunctival fibrovascular tissue was congested and hypertrophic; therefore, the wound appeared red, although the graft was flat and in place

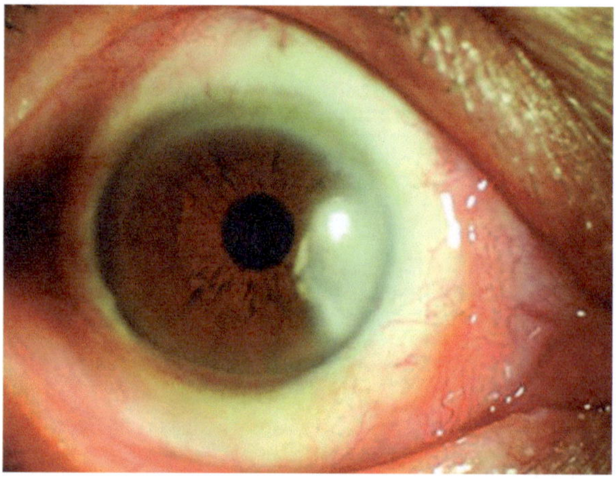

Fig. 8.28 Corneal degeneration and conjunctival dam-like changes. The original pterygium growth area on the nasal cornea was grey and degenerated, and the conjunctiva near the limbus was flat and was not congested; however, the semilunar plica was hypertrophic, and the junction area developed a red dam-like structure

3. Due to an overly small size or shrinkage of the graft, the original white area of the eye appears red (Fig. 8.27);
4. The graft is too large, causing the conjunctiva to be loose; and
5. If the hypertrophic semilunar plica is not resected or the subconjunctival pterygium tissue near the lacrimal caruncle is not radically removed, significant scarring at the graft and its junction site can result in a dam-like morphological change that affects cosmetic appearance (Fig. 8.28).

Preventive measures:

The corneal surface should be cleared as much as possible to restore smoothness. If obvious subpterygium corneal degeneration is observed prior to surgery, the patient and the family should be warned and mentally prepared about poor cosmetic outcomes. During surgery, the resected range for removing the degenerated conjunctiva and the size of the graft should not be too small, the hypertrophic semilunar plica should also be excised, and the nasal subconjunctival fibrovascular tissue near the lacrimal caruncle should be cleared to ensure even alignment between the conjunctival graft and the nasal conjunctiva.

Treatments:

Subpterygium corneal degeneration generally does not involve the pupillary area; hence, it can be left untreated if it does not significantly affect vision. Patients who have high cosmetic requirements can be performed partial lamellar keratoplasty. Poor conjunctival appearance after surgery does not need to be treated as long as it does not cause pterygium recurrence or functional restriction. Patients who have high cosmetic requirements can perform scar-removing surgery in combination with conjunctival flap autografting, and they can also undergo amniotic membrane transplantation if the defect is too large.

References

1. Huchzermeyer C, Gatzioufas Z, Kruse FE, et al. Treatment of severe recurrent symblepharopterygium: combined ipsilateral autologous limbus and homologous amniotic membrane transplantation. Der Ophthalmologe: Zeitschrift der Deutschen Ophthalmologischen Gesellschaft. 2014;9(111):839–45.
2. Natasha S. Assessing the quality of ophthalmic anesthesia. J Clin Anesth. 2015;4(27):285–9.
3. Ascaso FJ, Peligero J, Longás J, et al. Regional anesthesia of the eye, orbit, and periocular skin. Clin Dermatol. 2015;33(2):227–33.
4. Xia Q, Zhi H, Shen DA. Clinical analysis of the diplopia and strabismus after ophthalmic surgeries. Chin J Ophthalmol. 2003;39(12):727.
5. Hui-Ya F. The efficacy of fascial granuloma excision with conjunctival autografting after pterygium surgery. Graefes Arch Clin Exp Ophthalmol. 2018;10(256):1933–8.
6. Ahn SJ. Clinical features, predisposing factors, and treatment outcomes of scleritis in the Korean population. Korean J Ophthalmol. 2010;24(6):331–5.
7. Malik S, Khan MS, Basit I. Comparison of primary versus recurrent pterygium after intralesional 5-fluorouracil. J Pak Med Assoc. 2016;66(5):559–62.
8. Esquenazi S. Autogenous lamellar scleral graft in the treatment of scleral melt after pterygium surgery. Graefes Arch Clin Exp Ophthalmol. 2007;245(12):1869–71.
9. Wu H, Lin Z, Yang F, et al. Meibomian gland dysfunction correlates to the tear film instability and ocular discomfort in patients with pterygium. Sci Rep. 2017;7:45115.
10. Portoghese P. From models to molecules: opioid receptor dimers, bivalent ligands, and selective opioid receptor probes. J Med Chem. 2007;32(14):2259–69.
11. Ji-Eun L. Methicillin-resistant Staphylococcus aureus sclerokeratitis after pterygium excision. Cornea. 2007;6(26):744–6.
12. Peponis V, Rosenberg P, Chalkiadakis S, et al. Fungal scleral keratitis and endophthalmitis following pterygium excision. Eur J Ophthalmol. 2009;19(3):478.
13. Naser SA. Risk factors for pterygium recurrence after limbal-conjunctival autografting: a retrospective, single-centre investigation. Jpn J Ophthalmol. 2018;62(3):349–56.
14. Garg P, Sahai A, Shamshad M, et al. A comparative study of preoperative and postoperative changes in corneal astigmatism after pterygium excision by different techniques. Indian J Ophthalmol. 2019;67(7):1036–9.

MIX
Papier aus verantwortungsvollen Quellen
Paper from responsible sources
FSC® C105338

If you have any concerns about our products,
you can contact us on
ProductSafety@springernature.com

In case Publisher is established outside the EU,
the EU authorized representative is:
Springer Nature Customer Service Center GmbH
Europaplatz 3, 69115 Heidelberg, Germany

Printed by Libri Plureos GmbH
in Hamburg, Germany